10 Questions about

The Full Plate Diet™

1. **There are a lot of diet books, so what's special about this one?**
It's based on a simple, powerful concept—dietary fiber. "What Mom always told us to eat—fruits, vegetables, and other healthy foods."

2. **So, what about meat? Can I continue to eat meat on this diet?**
Sure, just eat your vegetables first. You'll understand why later.

3. **How does The Full Plate Diet work?**
Fiber fills you up and you'll eat fewer calories. Fewer calories means you lose weight. The beauty of The Full Plate Diet is you don't have to count calories—they take care of themselves.

4. **If this program is about fiber, does the food taste good?**
It's the best-tasting food you've ever eaten. Seriously.

5. **Can I begin the diet without making a lot of changes?**
Yes, the key is adding more fiber foods to what you already eat. We will show you how easy it is.

6. **Is there any research that supports the diet?**
Lots of medical research supports fiber as a proven way to lose weight and stay healthy.

7. **How much and how fast can I lose weight?**
Weight loss is the result of eating fewer calories than you burn. How much and how fast you lose is up to you.

8. **Why is this better than other diets I've tried?**
Most diets are a quick-fix and each of them comes with a backlash. Because you're making small changes it's easier to stay on The Full Plate Diet.

9. **Can I keep shopping at my regular grocery store?**
Absolutely.

10. **Can I stay in my food budget?**
Good news! The Full Plate Diet will probably cost you less than you're currently spending on food.

ONE LAST QUESTION: You say, "Eat more fiber." How, exactly, do I do that?
It's easy, easy, easy. You'll find everything you need to know in this book.

Change how you think and you'll change your actions. Change your actions and you'll change your weight. Change your weight and you'll change how you look. Feeling better, living longer, and having fewer health problems are just added benefits you get for free.

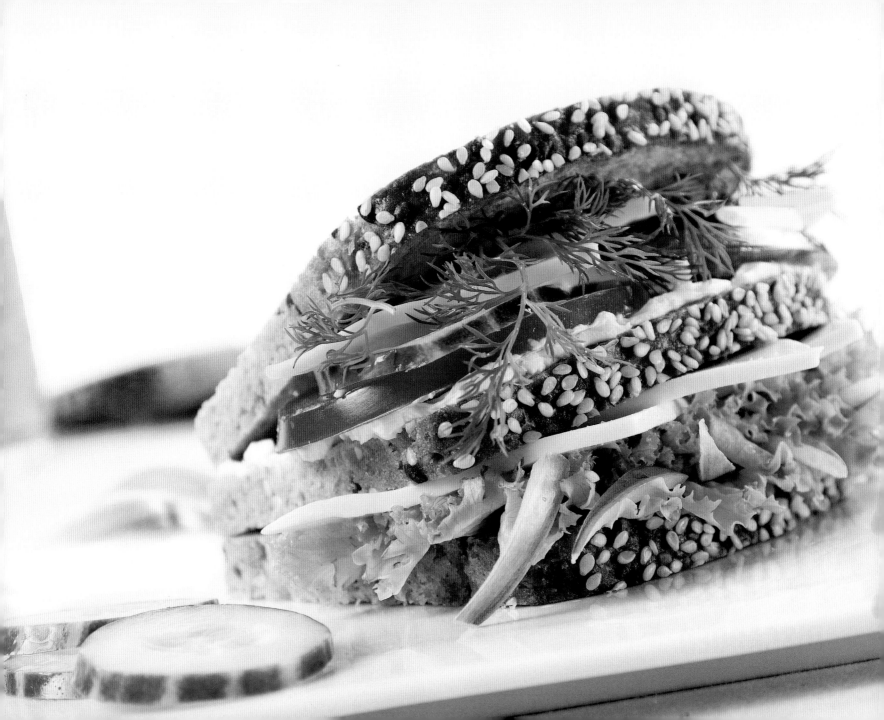

The Full Plate Diet

Slim Down, Look Great, Be Healthy!

Stuart A. Seale, M.D. • Teresa Sherard, M.D.
Diana Fleming, Ph.D., LDN

Bard Press

Austin, Texas

The Full Plate Diet™: Slim Down, Look Great, Be Healthy!
Printed by RR Donnelley in China

Bard Press
5275 McCormick Mtn. Dr.
Austin, TX 78734
512-266-2112, fax 512-266-2749
ray@bardpress.com
www.bardpress.com

This book contains the opinions and ideas of its authors. It is sold with the understanding that the authors and publisher are not engaged in rendering medical, health, or any other kind of personal or professional services to the reader. Accordingly, the information and dietary programs in this book are not intended to replace the services of trained medical professionals or be a substitute for medical advice, such as a dietary regimen that may have been prescribed by your physician. You should consult your physician or other competent health care professional before adopting any of the suggestions in this book or drawing inferences from it. While dietary changes may be helpful in the long run, they can also influence medication requirements. If you are currently taking diuretics, insulin, or oral diabetes medication, consult your physician before starting any diet recommended in this book. In addition, some individuals with long-standing diabetes may have already developed kidney damage, and in such cases a high-fiber diet could actually result in a dangerous buildup of potassium in the body. Individuals with kidney disease should have their dietary programs monitored by their physician. The authors and publisher specifically disclaim all responsibility for any liability, loss, or risk, personal or otherwise, which is incurred as a consequence, directly or indirectly, of the use and application of any of the contents of this book. Mention of specific companies, organizations, or authorities in this book does not imply endorsement by the authors or publisher, nor does mention of specific companies, organizations, or authorities imply that they endorse this book, its authors, or the publisher.

ISBN 13-digit 978-1-885167-71-2, 10-digit 1-885167-71-7

Library of Congress Cataloging-in-Publication Data

Seale, Stuart A.
 The full plate diet : slim down, look great, be healthy! / by Stuart A. Seale,
Teresa Sherard, and Diana Fleming.
    p. cm.
  Includes index.
  ISBN 978-1-885167-71-2
 1. Reducing diets. 2. Fiber in human nutrition. I. Sherard, Teresa. II. Fleming, Diana.
III. Title.

  RM222.2.S388 2010
  613.2'5—dc22
                      2009032035

Authors may be contacted at:
Lifestyle Center of America
4205 Goddard Youth Camp Rd.
Sulphur, OK 73086
1-800-596-5480
www.FullPlateDiet.org

Credits
Editor: Jeff Morris
Managing Editor: Sherry Sprague
Production Editor: Deborah Costenbader
Proofreader: Luke Torn
Indexer: Linda Webster
Cover Design: Hespenheide Design
Text Design & Production: Hespenheide Design
Photography: credits listed on page 152

Table of Contents

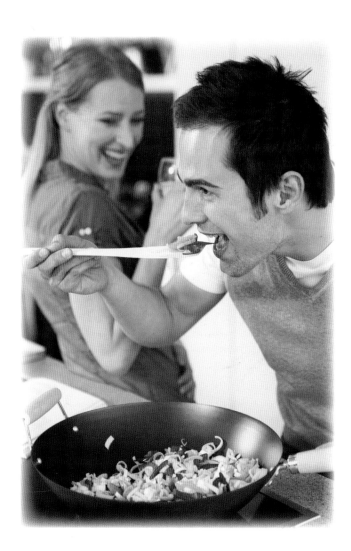

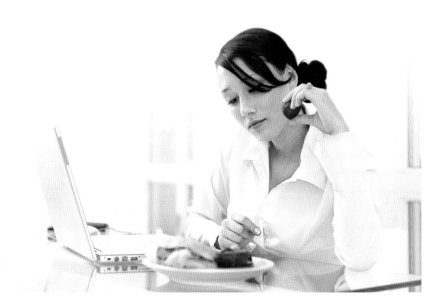

PART I

The Big Idea

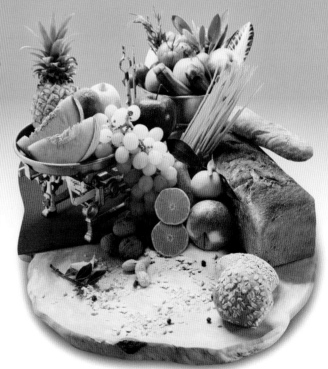

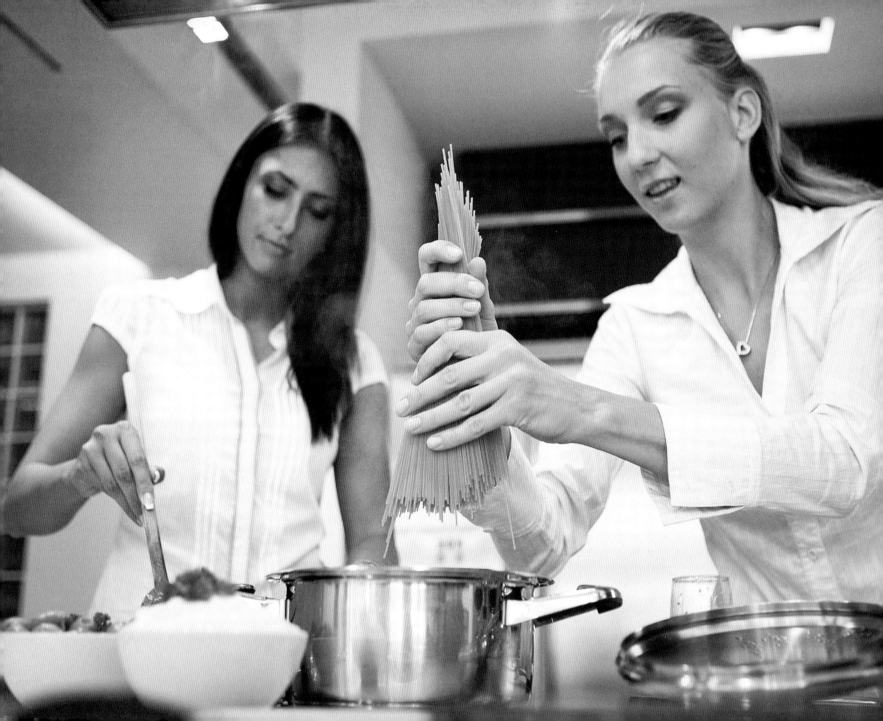

CHAPTER ONE

The Full Plate Concept

Fiber is suddenly hip. Grandma, it turns out, was just ahead of her time.

—Health & Nutrition Letter
Tufts University
February 2009

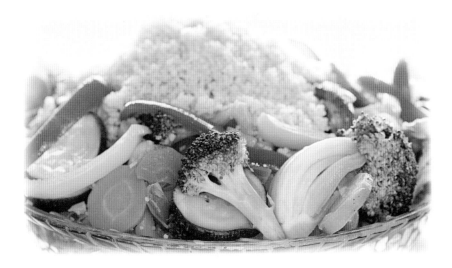

Fiber and Calories

Dietary fiber makes you feel full. Add fiber to your meals and you'll eat fewer calories. Consume fewer calories than you burn and you'll lose weight. It's that simple.

When most people think of fiber, they think of "roughage," like bran. Although insoluble dietary fiber is important, you also need soluble fiber. Both types of fiber are found in fruits, vegetables, whole grains, beans, nuts, and seeds.

The National Weight Control Registry tells us that 98% of the people who lost their target weight (an average of 66 pounds)—and kept it off long term—decreased their food intake to lose the weight. The Registry clearly indicates that a reduced-calorie diet is the way to maintain weight loss.

So do you want to eat tiny portions or a full plate? The only thing that matters is how many calories you consume.

Fiber contains no calories but it makes you feel full. Since fruits, vegetables, whole grains, beans, and nuts have lots of fiber and are easy to find, sustainable weight loss is simply a matter of buying healthy foods in the produce section of your grocery store, selecting the best products off the shelf, ordering the right foods on the menu, and not eating unless you are hungry.

Want to eat tiny portions or a full plate?

Your Diet Choices

You have lots of choices when choosing a diet.

Right to Your Front Door

Brand-name programs sell you packaged food and ship it to you every month. Do you really want to do this for the rest of your life? The day you quit mailing them checks will be the day you start gaining back all the weight you lost.

Big on Bacon & Steak

High-protein diets give you no limits on bacon, steak, and other fatty foods. But high protein means high cholesterol. Your eyes say yes but your heart says no. High protein = low health. Your body needs the vitamins, minerals, antioxidants, and phytochemicals that can be found only in fruits, vegetables, beans, nuts, and seeds.

Fad of the Month

Gimmick diets are everywhere—the grapefruit diet, the cabbage soup diet, the lemonade diet, the Hollywood diet, the chicken soup diet, even the Russian Air Force diet. How many of these have you tried? Did any of them work? More important, were you able to keep the pounds off?

Magic Pill

Infomercial producers have made millions of dollars selling ephedra, hoodia, green tea extract, and other "fat-burner" and "fat-blocker" pills to an anxious public. Ian K. Smith, M.D., dedicated himself to studying these products in extreme detail, then his findings were reported in *Time* magazine: "There are no shortcut pills to a leaner body."

Full Plate

The Full Plate Diet is easy, cheap, healthy, satisfying, sustainable—and most important, it works.

Harvard Study

The more fiber you eat, the more weight you'll lose. The less fiber you eat, the less weight you'll lose.

When Walter Willett, M.D., and his colleagues at the Harvard School of Public Health studied nearly 75,000 women over a 12-year period, one thing was obvious: the women who ate whole-grain fiber weighed less than the women who did not.

By stimulating the release of certain intestinal hormones, fiber promotes a feeling of satisfaction earlier in the meal. Fiber also slows the emptying of the stomach, prolonging that sense of fullness. As a result, fiber helps you eat less. It also slows the digestion and absorption of starches. This allows your body to break down dietary fats instead of storing them.

T. Colin Campbell, Ph.D., (author of *The China Study* and professor emeritus at Cornell University), Dean Ornish, M.D., and the National Heart, Lung, and Blood Institute have also published studies that demonstrate the power of fiber to facilitate weight loss. In addition, our 50 years of combined clinical practice, treating thousands of patients, has shown The Full Plate Diet to be the easiest and most sustainable way to get trim, feel great, and regain health. Weight loss of 5 to 10 pounds in the first month and 50 to 75 pounds after one year are not uncommon for those who follow our recommendations—without hunger or feelings of deprivation.

Why Diets Fail

Feeling full is due to food weight and volume, not calories. If you eat a meal high in calories, you can gain weight regardless of whether or not you feel full. If your idea of a diet is to keep eating those same high-calorie foods, only less of them, you'll feel deprived and probably won't succeed.

Most diets fail because they ask you to eat smaller portions and weights of food instead of changing the kinds of foods you're eating. Increase the amount of fiber in your diet and you'll have less room for the concentrated, high-calorie foods that make you overweight. It's as simple as that.

The more fiber you eat, the more weight you'll lose

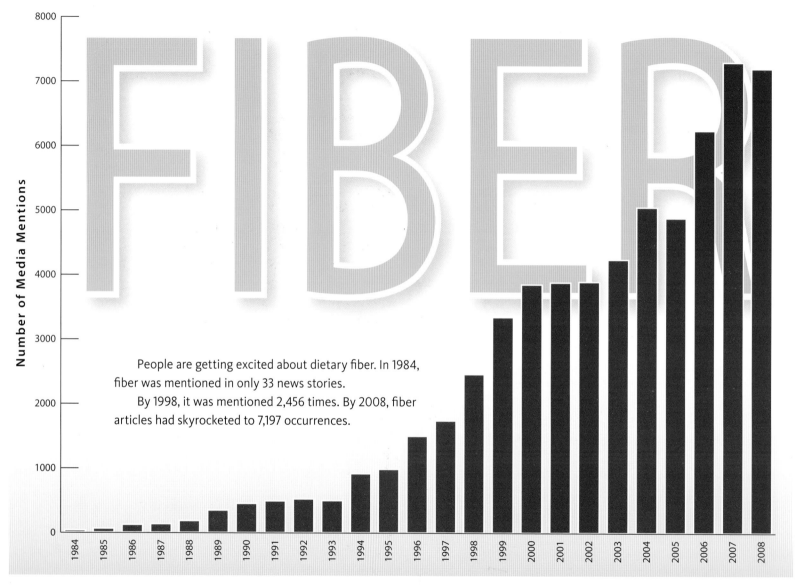

People are getting excited about dietary fiber. In 1984, fiber was mentioned in only 33 news stories.

By 1998, it was mentioned 2,456 times. By 2008, fiber articles had skyrocketed to 7,197 occurrences.

Nexis search of newspapers, newswire and press releases, aggregate news sources, industry trade press, magazines and journals, and news transcripts

Fiber has become the Next Big Thing in nutrition

The *Health & Nutrition Letter* from Tufts University for February 2009 contained a special report on fiber:

> Fiber—it's not just for Grandma anymore. Long the butt of jokes and hopelessly "un-hip," fiber has become the Next Big Thing in nutrition as Americans become more aware of its health benefits beyond battling constipation. A recent U.S. Department of Agriculture (USDA) survey found that dietary fiber information is the only labeling component to have seen an increase in use by U.S. consumers over the past decade.

Another indicator of the importance of fiber is the attention being paid to it by the food companies with the largest research divisions. Have you noticed how many new high-fiber packaged food products have been added to the shelves in recent months?

Kellogg's, Quaker Oats, General Mills, and Proctor & Gamble are just a few of the companies offering new products with added fiber. In addition, a number of other product categories have added fiber recently as well. Take a look in the dairy case of your local grocery store and you'll find high-fiber yogurt and high-fiber soymilk!

People are waking up to the power of fiber.

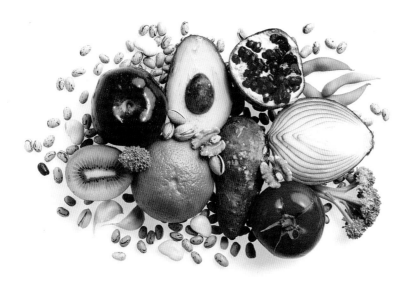

Twinkies, Twinkies Everywhere

The State of American Nutrition

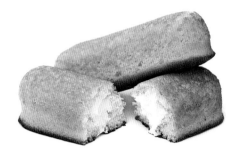

1. Americans eat more than 500 million Twinkies per year. Chicago is "the Twinkie capital of the world," gobbling down 27 million Twinkies annually. There is no fiber in a Twinkie.

2. Each year Americans drink an average of 490 12-ounce soft drinks. There's almost ¼ cup of sugar in a can of regular soda.

3. 34% of Americans are obese, with 33% being "overweight" and only 33% at normal weight. Only 5% of persons aged 12 to 19 were obese in 1976. Today it's 18%.

4. In the 1800s, the average American consumed only 10 pounds of sugar per year. Today it's 158 pounds. There is no fiber in sugar.

5. The U.S. is the fattest country in the world. Mexico is second, the U.K. third.

6. Obesity can shorten your life by 10 years. In 2000, obesity accounted for 400,000 American deaths, up from 300,000 in 1990.

7. Obesity will soon surpass tobacco as the leading cause of cancer in America.

8. American health care expenditures totaled $2.4 trillion in 2007, equal to 17% of the gross domestic product (GDP), rising at twice the rate of inflation.

9. The number of children who took pills for type 2 diabetes more than doubled from 2002 to 2005. Type 2 diabetes is closely linked to obesity. An estimated one out of every three children born in 2000 will develop type 2 diabetes.

10. Texas is the least healthy state, with Tennessee and South Carolina not far behind. Vermont is the healthiest state, with Hawaii and New Hampshire following.

For the sources of this information and other interesting facts about the American diet, go to **www.FullPlateDiet.org**.

CHAPTER TWO

The Big Health Benefits

If you have health, you probably will be happy, and if you have health and happiness, you have all the wealth you need, even if it is not all you want.

—Elbert Hubbard

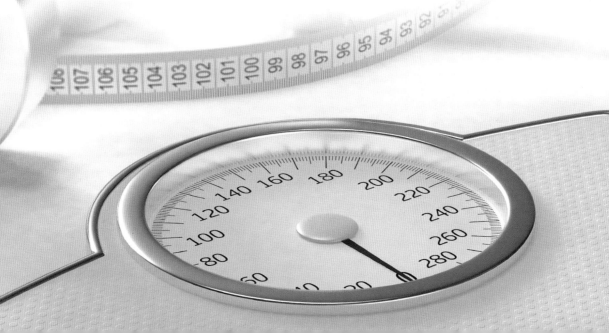

Medical researchers are among the strongest supporters of a high-fiber diet. The Institute of Medicine, the American Heart Association, the American Dietetic Association, and the American Diabetes Association all recommend that you increase your intake of dietary fiber. In addition to helping you lose weight and stay slim, The Full Plate Diet gives you these advantages (all supported by scientific research):

1. Heart Attack and Stroke? Fiber Lowers Your Risk

Consuming plant-based foods (fruits, vegetables, nuts, beans, and whole grains) is associated with a significantly lower risk of heart attack and stroke—up to 40% lower. What is it about these foods that protects you? Dietary fiber, antioxidants, phytochemicals, omega-3 fatty acids, potassium, and low sodium—all of which you will find in The Full Plate Diet.

2. Cancer? The Full Plate Diet Fights It

Fruit and vegetable consumption has a preventive effect for cancers of the stomach, esophagus, lung, oral cavity and pharynx, endometrium, pancreas, and colon. Vegetables and fruits protect against cancer by giving your body a rich supply of vitamins, minerals, antioxidants, and phytochemicals.

Doctors estimate that 30–40% of all cancers could have been prevented by lifestyle and dietary measures alone.

Lab experiments have shown that naturally occurring substances in The Full Plate Diet serve as dietary antimutagens. This means they reduce or interfere with substances that cause genetic mutation. It is believed that cancer is a disease caused by an accumulation of mutations in a cell.

More fruits and vegetables = more antimutagens = less cellular mutation = lower risk of cancer.

3. Diabetes? Fiber Controls the Sugar

"Based on current definitions, diabetes now affects an estimated 24.1 million people in the United States, an increase of more than 3 million in just 2 years. Another

Thirty to forty percent of all cancers could have been prevented by lifestyle and dietary measures alone

57 million people in the U.S. have pre-diabetes . . . which raises short-term absolute risk of type 2 diabetes 5- to 6-fold, and in some populations this may be even higher."—The American College of Endocrinology

In other words, 1 in 10 Americans currently have diabetes and indications are that this ratio will soon be 1 in 4. The rise of diabetes in America is due to the modern American diet creating an epidemic of obesity. Being overweight or obese can increase your risk of developing diabetes by up to 40 times.

Fiber reduces the risk of diabetes. The sugar spikes that trigger the pancreas to produce insulin are reduced by soluble fiber. Additionally, sugars are metered into the bloodstream more slowly when the digestive tract contains soluble fiber.

Eat more fiber. Your pancreas will thank you.

4. Lung Problems? Fiber Lets You Breathe Again

Emphysema, chronic bronchitis, and asthma are becoming more common as obesity rises in the U.S.

Obesity contributes to restricted breathing by placing excess weight on the chest and diaphragm. The problem increases as weight increases, especially if that weight is concentrated in the abdomen. Simply put, weight loss improves lung function.

The lung diseases mentioned above are all associated with inflammation, so a diet high in phytochemicals with anti-inflammatory properties can be extremely helpful. Phytochemicals are specialized

The rise of diabetes in America is due to the modern American diet

chemicals produced by plants to help them fight fungus and plant diseases. They have proven beneficial to humans as well. Berries are powerful fighters of inflammation, especially blueberries and strawberries.

Breathe easy on The Full Plate Diet.

5. Sleep Apnea? Lose Weight and Rest Easy

Losing weight reduces the symptoms of obstructive sleep apnea. The Division of Endocrinology at the University of Colorado, Denver, determined that "in severely obese patients, even moderate weight loss (approximately 10%) boasts substantial benefit in terms of the severity of sleep-disordered breathing and sleep dynamics."

Sleep soundly on The Full Plate Diet.

6. Digestive Complaints? Fiber Calms the Storm

If you're battling chronic constipation, you need plenty of high-fiber foods. "Fiber is a stool regulator, a stool normalizer," says Paul McNeely, M.D., a gastroenterologist at the Ochsner Health System in New Orleans.

Fiber also works as a diarrhea treatment. "Fiber can't work miracles," McNeely says, "but if you have a loose stool, a lot of excess liquid in the stool, the fiber in your colon will absorb and firm up the stool, which definitely helps diarrhea."

The best foods are unprocessed whole-plant foods

7. Heartburn? Throw Away the Tums

Heartburn can be caused by the foods you eat. Fatty foods increase heartburn; dietary fiber reduces it. The Full Plate Diet lets you win both ways. Heartburn is your body's way of telling you it needs more soluble fiber. Listen to your gut.

Abdominal cavity pressure goes up as you gain weight, pushing stomach acid up into the lower esophagus where it doesn't belong. This creates a feeling commonly known as heartburn or acid reflux. Lose weight and your symptoms will probably disappear.

8. Colon Problems? Fiber Fights 'Em

Inflammatory bowel disease involving either the small or large intestine can result in pain, blood in the stool, diarrhea, and possible malabsorption of nutrients. Soluble fiber is digested by colon bacteria to produce butyrate, a compound that reduces inflammation. Some foods naturally high in fiber have inflammation-reducing omega-3 fatty acids that stabilize inflammatory bowel disease, and low amounts of compounds that increase inflammation.

9. Joint Pain? Feel Free to Flex

Osteoarthritis is caused by inflammation and erosion of cartilage in the joints, especially the knees, back, hip, and hands. This destruction of cartilage is related to the production of cytokines by fat, as well as wear and tear on the joints. Weight loss can help in two ways. It (1) reduces mechanical stress and (2) lowers the level of cytokines. The result? A reduction in pain and disability and an increase in performance. Even small amounts of weight loss can yield pleasant results.

10. Fatigued? Tap Your Inner Child's Energy

Sugar and caffeine will give you a short jolt of energy followed by a crash. Not only does this crash feel bad, it's hard on the body. The best foods for long-lasting energy are unprocessed, whole-plant foods—fruits, vegetables, beans, and whole grains. The worst are those that have little fiber, such as processed plant foods and animal products—in other words, fast food and vending machine snacks. These convenience foods leave us overfed and undernourished.

Fiber foods deliver a wide array of the micronutrients your body requires to function at full capacity. The Full Plate Diet gives you the nutrition you need to feel young again.

11. Too Tired to Tango?

Male sexual function improves with weight loss. Sexual inventory scores improve in all categories, including sexual drive, erectile and ejaculatory function, and sexual satisfaction.

Women's scores likewise improve following weight loss. Women experience feelings of sexual attractiveness, sexual desire, a willingness to be seen undressed, and enjoyment of sexual activity.

Both men and women report an overall increase in the frequency, quality, and enjoyment of sex following weight loss. As body image improves, there is an increase in the initiation of sexual intercourse, decreased sexual inhibition, increased sexual enjoyment, and increased frequency of orgasm.

Fiber is sounding better and better, isn't it?

Lose weight. Regain your sexuality.

Heartburn is your body's way of telling you it needs more soluble fiber

12. In Short: Live Longer, Live Better

There's ample evidence that a reduced-calorie diet can increase your longevity, but only if you consume sufficient vitamins, minerals, and phytonutrients. In other words, consume the highest-quality, most nutrient-packed foods possible—those found in The Full Plate Diet.

Caloric restriction works on three different levels: (1) As food intake decreases, metabolism slows down and the free radicals that form as by-products of metabolism decrease as well. This is good. (2) Less free radicals means less cellular damage and a lower likelihood of cancer and other diseases linked to free radicals. (3) Additionally, caloric restriction causes an increase in protective enzymes that counteract free radicals.

What all this means is that the fruits, vegetables, beans, nuts, and whole grains of The Full Plate Diet work to give you a longer, healthier life.

Besides, they taste great.

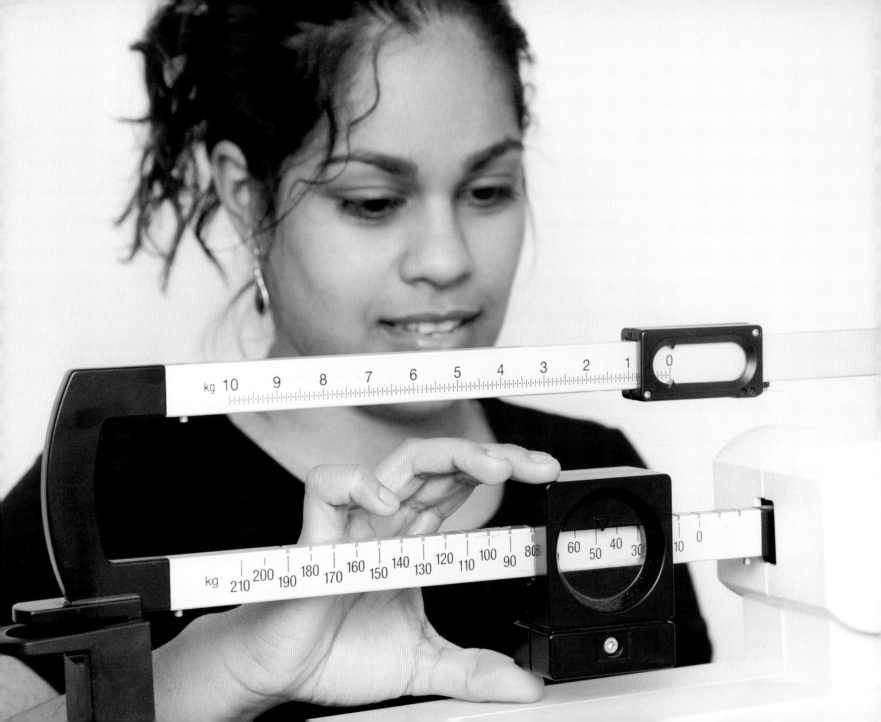

PART II

Getting Started

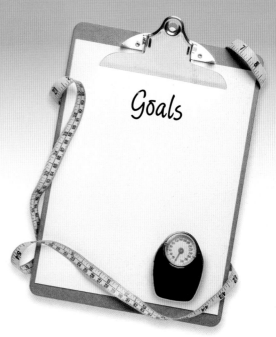

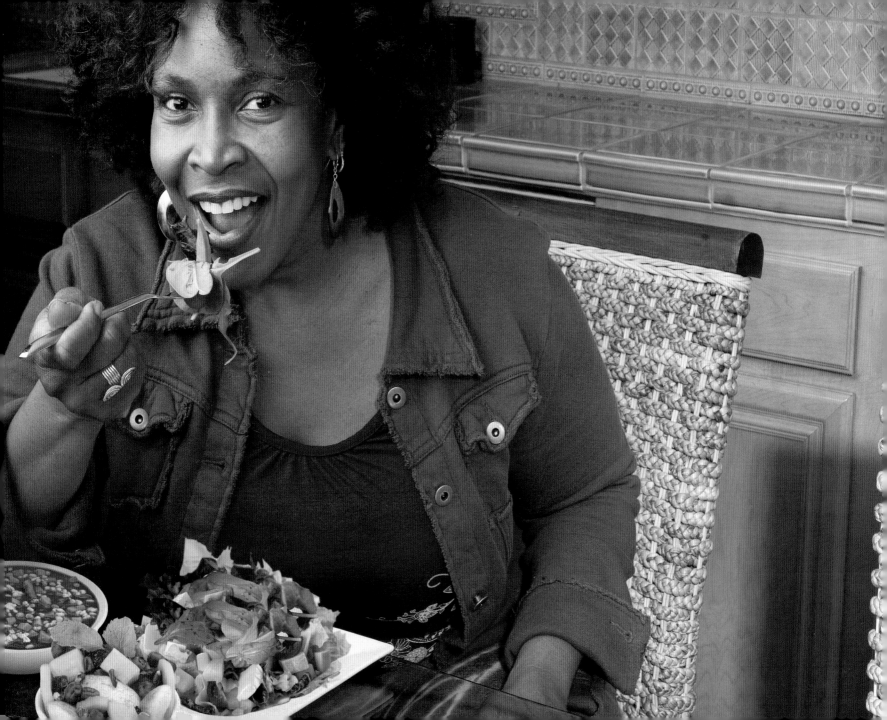

CHAPTER THREE

Starting Where You Are

You have brains in your head. You have feet in your shoes.

You can steer yourself in any direction you choose.

You're on your own. And you know what you know.

And YOU are the one who'll decide where to go.

—Dr. Seuss
Oh, the Places You'll Go!

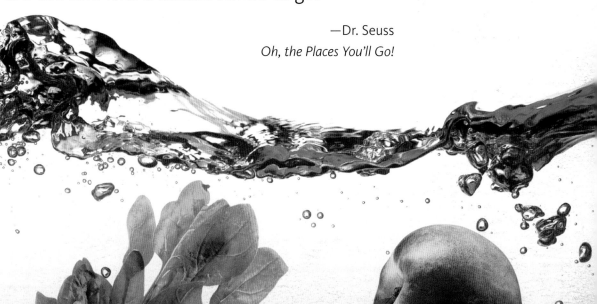

How Much Fiber Do You Eat?

If you eat a typical American diet, which consists of about 3 total servings per day of fruits and vegetables, little or no beans, and white or enriched bread and cereals, then you are probably consuming about 10 grams of fiber per day. That doesn't sound like much when you compare it to our recommendation of 40 or more grams per day, but The Full Plate Diet will make it easy for you to accomplish your goal. Just start with our recommendations for Stage One. The good news is that people who need to make the most changes also gain the most benefit, usually in the shortest period of time.

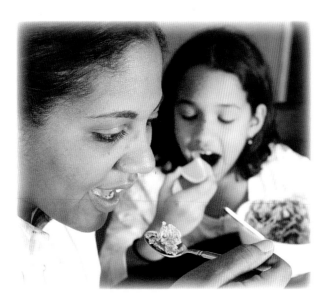

Many high-fiber foods are jumping with protein

Perhaps you eat more than 3 but less than 9 total servings per day of fruits and vegetables. Maybe you eat some beans and usually stick to whole-grain cereals and bread. That is good—you are probably getting closer to 20 grams of fiber per day—better than average, but still not quite enough. If you follow our advice for those in Stage Two, you will find it is easy to boost your fiber intake up to our recommendation, especially if you power-up the foods you are eating now with fiber-packed additions. See our Power Up section (part III) for ideas, then experiment on your own and develop Power Ups and Fiber Wheels that best fit your routine and preferences. In no time you will find your fiber intake going up, and your bathroom scale going down.

There may be some of you who eat 9 servings of fruits and vegetables per day, as well as beans and whole grains. Congratulations! You may be getting the 40 grams of fiber per day The Full Plate Diet recommends. You are in Stage Three, and likely will just need to fine-tune things a bit in order to start losing weight. For example, make sure you eat fiber foods at every meal and snack, and always eat fiber foods first. Eat fewer snacks between meals and during the four hours before bedtime. Gradually increase your physical activity. Become a nutrition detective and start paying attention to food labels. All of these actions will help you become, and maintain, a thinner, healthier you.

Want to have some fun and learn about how much fiber you eat in a day? Go to **www.FullPlateDiet.org/ fiber-calculator**, and check out the fiber calculator. It's easy to use—and you will also learn about which foods have high and low fiber.

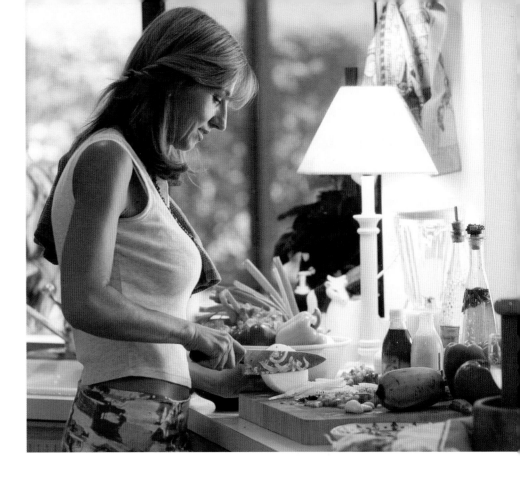

He can who thinks he can,
and he can't who thinks he can't.
This is an inexorable, indisputable law.

—Pablo Picasso

The Three Stages

The key to losing weight is to eat fewer calories than your body burns each day. Fiber foods fill you faster and contain fewer calories. This is how they help you reduce your intake of calorie-concentrated foods.

Here's what too often happens: You buy a diet book, excited about a new way to finally lose those extra pounds. Then you get it home and start to read lists of rules, do's and don'ts. There's no way you're ever going to be able to do this! A few months later, you give the book to Goodwill.

The good news about The Full Plate Diet is that it works even when you do it imperfectly.

You can improve how you look and feel without ever progressing past Stage One.

You just need to eat more fiber

Stage One

1. Eat more fiber foods.
2. Drink more water—at least 6 glasses a day.
3. Stop eating when you no longer feel hungry.

If Stage One is easy for you and you feel like pushing farther, faster, move to Stage Two:

Stage Two

1. Increase the fiber in your diet to new levels. Eat fiber foods at the beginning of every meal or snack.
2. Experiment with a wider variety of high-fiber foods.
3. Drink even more water, 8 to 10 glasses per day. (Your body needs more water when you eat more fiber.)

If you're that one-in-a-thousand person (seriously, it's about one in a thousand) who has the interest and the discipline to push an idea all the way to its limits, here's Stage Three:

Stage Three

1. Stabilize your fiber intake to a consistent 40+ grams each day.
2. Become a "label detective." Always learn what's in the food before you put it in your basket at the grocery store. You'll find all the information you need at **www.FullPlateDiet.org**.
3. Reduce your intake of meat and dairy products, as well as other foods that are high calorie, high fat, and low fiber.

Full Plate Payoffs

Like anything else, what you get from The Full Plate Diet depends entirely on what you put into it. We suggest you start slowly.

Here's what we don't want to happen: First week of January—New Year's resolution—get in shape. You put on your new track outfit and run 5 miles. The next morning you have so many aches and pains you can barely get out of bed. "It's just not worth it."

Okay, maybe you never did the New Year's thing. But did you ever sign up for a year's membership at a gym and then decide that you really didn't have the time? Here's our point: don't go nuts. In addition to losing weight, The Full Plate Diet has long-term health benefits, so it's important that you don't try to change so much, so fast, that you end up quitting.

Your long-term goal is to eat at least 40 grams of fiber a day. Some of our patients eat 45 grams or more. But if you move to these levels too quickly, your digestive system will complain in ways that neither you nor your friends will like.

The 40+ grams of fiber level will be reached when you're ready. If you're currently eating only 10 grams of fiber a day, it will probably take you at least a few weeks to get to 40 grams. If you're currently at 20 grams, you'll be at 40 much faster.

Don't go nuts

When you're ready, your long-term goal is to eat at least 40 grams of fiber a day

It's Not That Hard

You'll be surprised how easy it is to increase your fiber intake. You'll read about 55 of the best high-fiber foods in Chapter 5. In chapter 6 you'll learn how you can add high-fiber foods to what you already eat. You're going to be pleasantly surprised how many of these foods you like. You just need to eat more of them.

In the following chapter, you'll find several tips to help you be successful. People tell us it's not that hard to get started. For example, Joe Hamilton, a media analyst at a communications firm we hired before writing this book, was intrigued by what we were saying about fiber. He asked a few questions, got the basic idea—eat more fiber, drink more water, stop eating when you no longer feel hungry—and lost 90 lbs in 14 months. Joe dropped from a plump 280 to a movie star 190. For more personal examples, visit **www.FullPlateDiet.org**.

Exercise, of course, burns calories. Remember the study published by the National Weight Control Registry you read about in chapter 1? Losing weight is all about

Fiber helps you lose weight naturally

cutting calories, plain and simple. The beauty of The Full Plate Diet is that increasing your fiber intake helps you lose weight naturally because you're consuming fewer calories. Even if you don't increase your exercise you still lose weight. Exercise will definitely help you burn calories faster, but again, it's up to you.

Your Eating Style: Busy, Busy, Busy

Did you ever see *Leave It to Beaver*? The Cleavers were the quintessential family of the 1950s. June Cleaver had dinner on the table every evening at precisely 5:30 for her husband, Ward, and her two boys, Wally and Beaver. They sat down and ate together every evening as a family. And of course June Cleaver vacuumed the house every day wearing high heels and pearls. Things have changed a bit, haven't they?

Today's June Cleaver juggles work and a family. Like all of us, she's on the go. Like her, we can only dream of everyone sitting down to eat at the same time. The good news is that it's easy to incorporate high fiber into a busy life.

Chapter 6 has suggestions of high-fiber foods you, the kids, and your significant other can eat to replace those foods that have low or no fiber. You'll also find Power Ups and *very* simple Fiber Wheels to get you started.

On the Go—Eating Out

Lots of us frequently eat at casual and fast-food restaurants. Finding more fiber in these situations can be a challenge, but menus are changing and most restaurants are happy to accommodate requests for items not on the menu. In chapter 7 you'll find suggestions for eating fiber at your workplace, in restaurants, and on the road.

Already into Food and Nutrition?

If you've been reading about nutrition, you know the experts are already singing the praises of fiber. The Full Plate Diet, with fiber as its main theme, will help you attain that elusive next level. Take the opportunity to experiment and enjoy the fiber path to weight loss and a healthy lifestyle.

If you're enjoying retirement or working from home you can eat what you want, when you want, so you've got total freedom to put The Full Plate Diet to work.

Most of us move in and out of these eating styles. Sometimes, we're busy, busy, busy and on the go and eating out. Occasionally we're at home—weekends, vacations, holidays—giving us more time to experiment with high-fiber meals.

"Hey, Authors! What About Protein?"

If you're worried about not getting enough protein—relax. All fiber-rich foods contain protein, and many are just jumping with it. It's virtually impossible to eat a high-fiber diet and fail to get enough protein. The Full Plate Diet is the most nutritious diet a person can eat. Your body is going to love you for it.

If you really want to dig into the details, go to **www.FullPlateDiet.org**, where you'll find mountains of interesting facts and all the latest scientific research.

Are You Ready?

The Full Plate Diet is a powerful way to lose weight. But no matter how effective the diet may be, your results will depend on your willingness to change some of your old habits into healthier ones. The fact that you're taking the time to read this book means you're at least thinking about making changes. You may be anxious to get going. Hopefully this is the case, but a word of caution is in order: When a change of behavior is undertaken without adequate preparation, failure will follow more often than not. This leads to discouragement and a belief that the diet itself was at fault.

We want to help you avoid that outcome.

You get enjoyment from your habits, even the problematic ones. If this weren't the case, you wouldn't have the habits. You want to lose weight, but you also want to continue the behaviors that caused you to gain the weight. If you get more satisfaction from your old habits than what you secretly believe you'll get from losing weight, this diet is going to fail.

When you are convinced—deep in your heart—that losing weight and being healthy are more important than what you're giving up, then you're ready for action and you will likely succeed.

We've included a Readiness Assessment from the work of James Prochaska, Ph.D., to help you determine if you're ready for change.

When you are convinced that losing weight is more important than what you're giving up, then you're ready for action and you will likely succeed

> Things do not change; we change

—Henry David
Thoreau
Walden

Readiness Assessment

Take a minute to assign a score (1–5) to each of the following 16 statements. This is important.

If you don't want to write in the book, grab a sheet of paper and write the numbers 1 to 16 in a vertical column, then read the 16 statements below and assign a score to each question number.

Please assign 1, 2, 3, 4, or 5 to each of the 16 statements below:

1 = not important   **2** = slightly important
3 = somewhat important   **4** = quite important
5 = extremely important

- [ ] **1.** Some people would think less of me if I changed.
- [ ] **2.** I would be healthier if I changed.
- [ ] **3.** Changing would take a lot of time.
- [ ] **4.** Some people would feel better about me if I changed.
- [ ] **5.** I'm concerned I might fail if I tried to change.
- [ ] **6.** Changing would make me feel better about myself.
- [ ] **7.** Changing takes a lot of effort and energy.
- [ ] **8.** I would function better if I changed.
- [ ] **9.** I would have to give up some things I enjoy.
- [ ] **10.** I would be happier if I changed.
- [ ] **11.** I get some benefit from my current behavior.
- [ ] **12.** Some people would be better off if I changed.
- [ ] **13.** Some people benefit from my current behavior.
- [ ] **14.** I would worry less if I changed.
- [ ] **15.** Some people would be uncomfortable if I changed.
- [ ] **16.** Some people would be happier if I changed.

Crunching Your Numbers

Add up the total score you gave the odd-numbered statements, then do the same for the even-numbered ones.

If the total for the odd-numbered questions is 17 or below, and the even-numbered score is at least 28 or above, you're definitely ready to change and the likelihood of your success is high. If your odd-numbered total is higher than 17, or the even-numbered total is below 28, we recommend you proceed slowly with Stage One, and don't push further until you're certain you're ready. Your body won't change until your actions change. And your actions won't change until your thoughts have changed. You'll know when you're ready to move from Stage One to Stage Two.

Two Techniques for Getting Ready

1. Write a paragraph that describes what it's like to be overweight. Write another paragraph describing how different things will be when you're at your ideal weight. Read these paragraphs every day, even after

you have them memorized. Reading your own words is a powerful tool for change.

2. As you eat, imagine healthy foods immediately burning as fuel to produce energy. When tasting sweets or processed snacks, imagine them becoming fat and going to exactly the spot you'd most like to trim down. Your imagination is a powerful tool, and it wants to help you. Let it.

For more tips and techniques, go to **www.FullPlate Diet.org**.

Making the Commitment

If you're ready to begin The Full Plate Diet, there are some things you can do to accelerate your success. Again, these are optional. Go as far as you feel comfortable.

1. Take a look at I'M READY! on the next page. If you feel ready to go, sign your name. Little actions like this are known to deepen personal commitment.
2. If you're willing to announce your commitment and deepen your resolve, (1) go to **www.FullPlate Diet.org**, (2) click "I'M READY!" and (3) type in your name.
3. The page after I'M READY! is I'M GOING FOR IT! If you'd like to tell your family, friends, and co-workers what you're doing, this is an easy way to do it. Make as many copies as you want.
4. There are cut-out pages for I'M READY! and I'M GOING FOR IT! at the back of the book. You can put I'M READY! on your refrigerator door or near your bathroom mirror. Make as many copies as you want of both pages.

Why are we suggesting that you make a commitment in writing? You already know the answer. When we make a commitment in writing, even to ourselves, we increase the likelihood of following through. Yes, it sounds silly, but it works. When we announce our commitment to the world, and especially to people we care about, we heighten our desire to succeed. We want to show them we can do it.

On to chapter 4!

> If you feel ready to go, sign your name, put it on your refrigerator door, and tell your family, friends, and co-workers

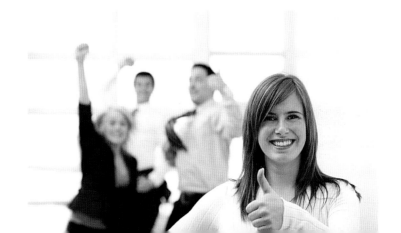

I'm Ready!

I've read the first 3 chapters in The Full Plate Diet. I like the concept and both payoffs—losing the pounds and better natural health. I'm ready to go.

I've read and understand the 3 things I need to do in Stage One:

1. Eat more fiber foods.
2. Drink more water—at least 6 glasses a day.
3. Stop eating when I no longer feel hungry.

I'm committed to making it work for me. I see a thinner me.

_____   _____

My Name   Date

I'm Going for It!

I'm going to make some conscious changes in the way I eat that will make a big difference in how I look and feel. I'm getting slim!

The Full Plate Diet is about eating foods I like, and making sure I eat a lot more foods with fiber—fruits, vegetables, beans, and whole grains.

I'm going to eat more fiber, drink more water, and stop eating when I am not hungry.

This is a long-term, sustainable lifestyle change that will give me energy and improve my health in many ways.

Expect me to start looking slimmer soon—and know that I'll be eating more fruits, vegetables, beans, and whole grains at every opportunity.

Wish me well.

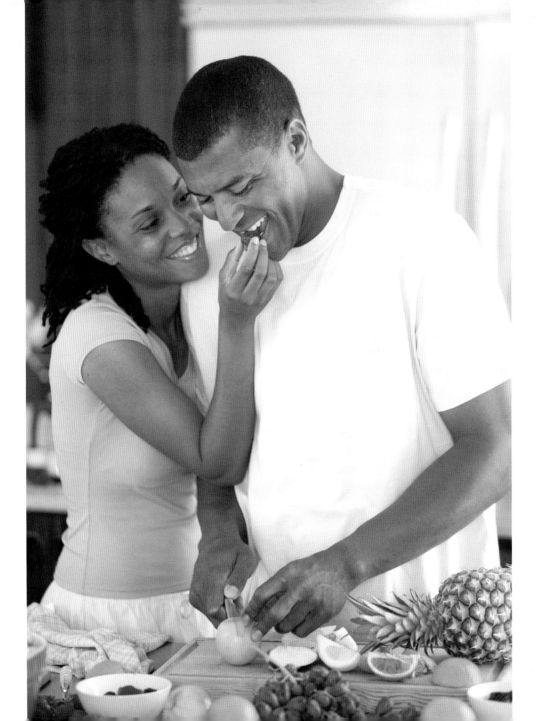

A table, a chair, a bowl of fruit and a violin; what else does a man need to be happy?

—Albert Einstein

CHAPTER FOUR

Getting Slimmer Happens One Pound at a Time

Never lose an opportunity of urging a practical beginning, however small, for it is wonderful how often in such matters the mustard-seed germinates and roots itself.

—Florence Nightingale

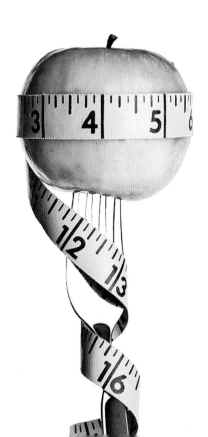

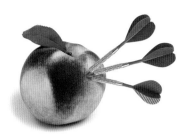

Set Your Goal

Millions of people wish they were thinner, but a wish is just a wish—on its own it doesn't do much.

Your first step is to set a weight-loss goal. Having a target weight in your mind—and on paper—increases the odds that you will be successful. Tape your number on your refrigerator door, your bathroom mirror, and other places where you can see it every day.

Now you need to set a second goal, a short-term goal, an immediate target. A long-term goal such as "lose 40 pounds in the next 12 months" can feel impossible when you're standing at the bottom of the mountain. Lower your sights. Losing 3 pounds this month seems much more achievable, doesn't it? When you've lost 3 pounds and have only 37 to go, that mountain doesn't seem quite so high.

If you don't achieve your short-term goal, set a new one! Just keep moving toward your long-term goal. Perfection is not required. Everyone misses the mark occasionally. The important thing is to keep moving ahead.

Don't set yourself up to fail. Losing 40 pounds in 2 months isn't a good goal. People who lose weight that quickly almost always gain it back. Set goals you can achieve. Achieving your short-term goal builds confidence and deepens your resolve. Three pounds at a time. Just 3 pounds. You can do it.

Now let's lose those first 3.

Find a Friend or Two, or Five

Some people find things easier to do in a group. Are you one of them? If so, tell your friends about The Full Plate Diet and see if they want to join you. They may be ready to make the commitment.

Think of your friends from high school or college, church or community organizations. Co-workers can make excellent partners in weight loss. You can also go online, using Facebook or other social media. Your friends don't all have to live in the same town.

A friend is someone who will share the experience, act as a sounding board, and offer encouragement and suggestions, as well as be an accountability partner.

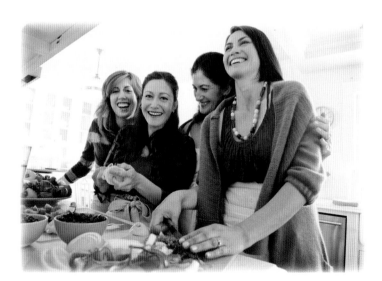

Support Along the Way

The three of us writing this book work for the Lifestyle Center of America, a non-profit organization whose only mission is to help people live longer, better, healthier lives.

Go to **www.FullPlateDiet.org** and you'll find a number of things we have created to assist you.

* A fiber calculator to help you determine your fiber starting point
* Encouraging success stories
* A message board to share your experience and learn from others
* Weekly tips will inspire new ways to make The Full Plate Diet work for you
* Insider Tip email provides weekly ideas along with exclusive diet nuggets directly in your Inbox

Weighing & Keeping a Log

If you have a good bathroom scale, that's all you need. If you weigh every day, be sure to weigh at the same time each day. Some people weigh less often, like once a week. Do whatever works for you. Joe Hamilton, the guy in chapter 3 who lost 90 pounds, weighed himself only 3 or 4 times during the first 14 months. Joe knew he was losing weight from the notches in his belt. That was enough for him.

Other people might like to keep a daily log, writing down their weight each day. This is an equally good idea. Different personality types respond to different forms of measurement and feedback. But if you choose to weigh yourself daily, it's important that you not get

discouraged when you don't lose weight for a few days. You might occasionally even gain a pound or two. The important thing is your trend over time. Looking at your daily numbers to find a 7- or 10-day average is a more accurate way to measure your progress. The battle isn't won in a day, a week, or even a month. You didn't add the weight that fast and you're not going to lose it that fast either.

But you can lose it faster than you gained it.

Exercise If You Want

You learned in chapter 1 that weight loss is all about calories. Exercise burns calories, so supplementing your diet with exercise will help. But you don't need to go to the gym. Just move more—take the stairs instead of the elevator. Park farther away when shopping. Always look for ways you can be more active.

Easy & Powerful Technique

Larry Wilson wrote an award-winning book, *Play to Win: Choosing Growth over Fear in Work and Life*. Larry has a marvelous technique for evaluating choices before taking action. You need to

* Stop
* Challenge
* Choose

when making a decision that will influence your weight.

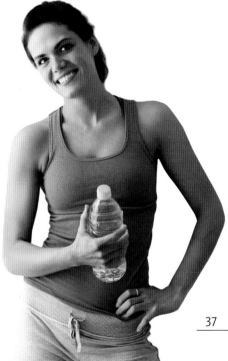

How Change Happens

1. Learn about the problem you're facing and how to overcome it.

   (Weight is gained when excess calories are consumed, and modern foods tend to be calorie-concentrated.)

2. Find out why you have gained weight and what will correct it.

   (You've been eating more calories than you burn.)

3. Analyze your past habits and determine how they should be changed.

   (You need to eat fewer calories. Foods high in fiber are filling, but low in calories.)

4. Gather reliable information.

   (You are doing this now, by reading this book.)

5. Rely on the support of others.

   (Seek out restaurants that serve healthy foods. Find a local health food store and talk to the staff—they live to help people new to healthy eating.)

6. Include your family and friends.

   (Recruit an accountability partner—someone you will allow to be openly honest with you.)

7. Think positive. You can do this!

   (Don't let yourself feel deprived when you choose not to eat calorie-concentrated foods. Be glad you have options. Millions of people have no options regarding what they eat. You're one of the lucky ones. You get to choose.)

8. Give yourself small rewards for making good choices.

   (You said no to the chocolate cake that contains no fiber, so go ahead and splurge on that pricey, exotic high-fiber fruit you saw at the market. A person who can say no to chocolate deserves a quart of perfect blackberries!)

> ## Try? There is no try. There is only do or not do.
>
> —Yoda
> *Star Wars:*
> *The Empire Strikes Back*

9. Create safe havens at home and work.

(Don't surround yourself with temptations. Instead of that bag of candy you keep in your desk, stash an apple or some almonds.)

10. Make good choices at the supermarket.

(Then it's easy to make good choices at mealtime.)

The people you love most are going to watch you become thinner, healthier, and happier. Your success is going to encourage them. You're not doing this for yourself alone.

The people you love will follow in your footsteps if only you'll lead the way.

Remember These 3 Things:

1. Eat more fiber foods.
2. Drink more water.
3. Stop eating when you no longer feel hungry.

Do these things and your weight will melt away.

Never eat more than you can lift.

—Miss Piggy

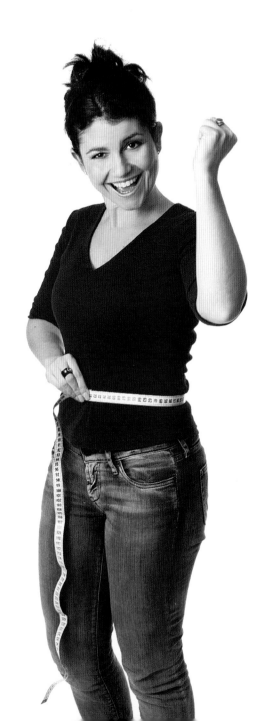

How different would your life be if you were at your ideal weight?

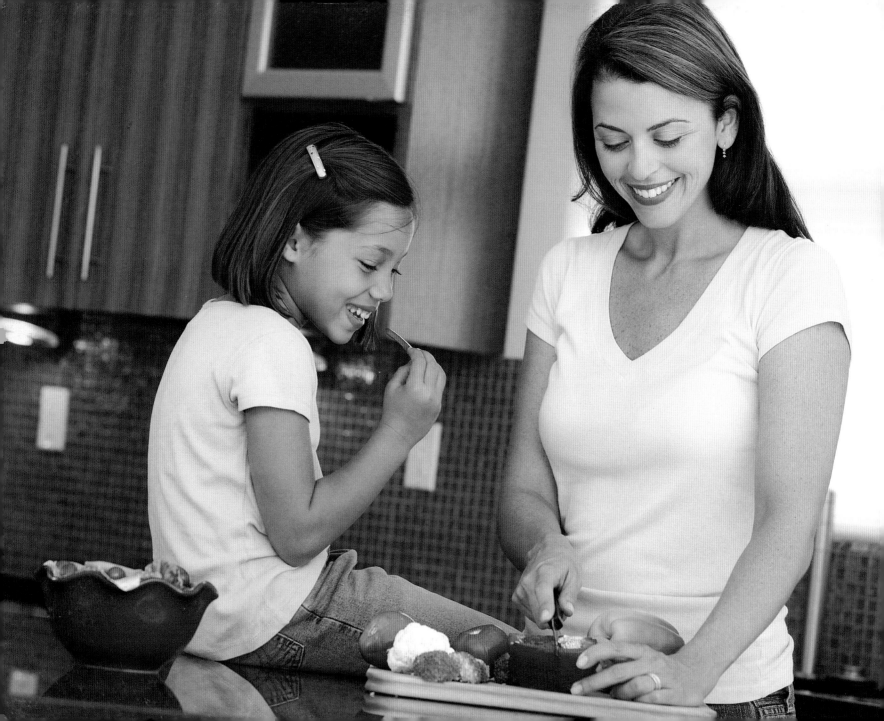

PART III

Power Fibers to Take the Pounds Off

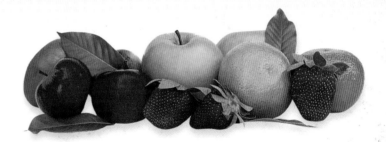

Things You Need to Know
About Chapter 5

Important things are sometimes disclosed on a "need to know" basis. The following things aren't particularly important, but we still think you need to know.

"Top 5" Lists

We used the following criteria to select the Top 5 food items in each of the 5 food categories:

1. How much fiber does the food contain?
2. How easy is the food to find?

That's why you'll find wonderful foods like papaya on the Honorable Mentions list instead of within the Top 5s. Although it's higher in fiber than 3 of the foods in the Top 5s, it's not as easy to find.

No Decimals

Nutritional information is rounded to the nearest whole number. As scientists, we would have felt better with the decimals in place, but the publisher just rolled his eyes and said, "Trust me."

Fun Facts

We want you to think about what you eat, so we dug up as many fun pieces of food trivia as we could find. If you think differently, you'll eat differently, and then you'll feel better and look *FABULOUS* .

Health Benefits

We highlighted a few of the health benefits you'll gain by eating high-fiber foods. Our goal is to increase your intake of these healthy foods—and speed your weight loss.

Nutrition Information

We chose the same format you'll find on food labels. A quick glance will give you information of importance and interest to you—carbohydrates, calories, sodium, saturated fat, etc. The USDA was our source for fiber grams for each food. The fiber grams may vary from product to product. If you want to check go to **www.nal.usda.gov/fnic/foodcomp/Data/SR17/wtrank/sr17a291.pdf**.

Like we said

at the top of the page, these things aren't particularly important, we just thought you needed to know. *Now if only the publisher would let us include those decimals . . .*

CHAPTER FIVE

Top 5s & Honorable Mentions

Food can look beautiful, taste exquisite, smell wonderful, make people feel good, bring them together, inspire romantic feelings.

—Rosamond Richardson

Top 5 Fruits

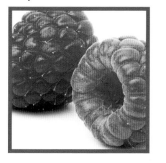

Top 5 Vegetables

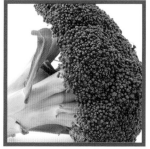

Top 5 Beans

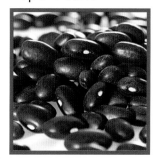

Top 5 Nuts & Seeds

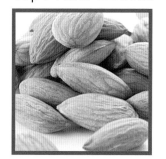

Top 5 Grains

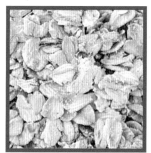

Top 5 Fruits for Your Diet

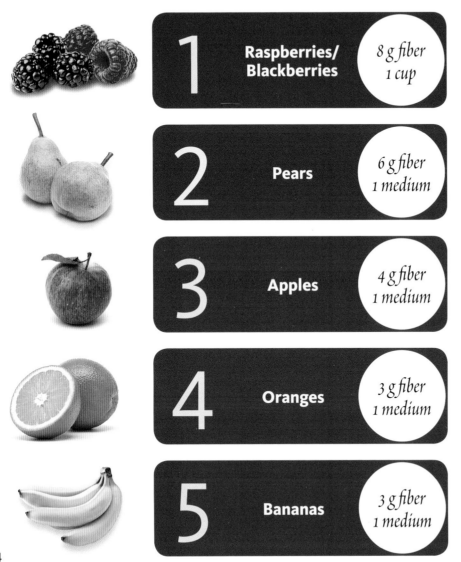

1 **Raspberries/ Blackberries** — *8 g fiber 1 cup*

2 **Pears** — *6 g fiber 1 medium*

3 **Apples** — *4 g fiber 1 medium*

4 **Oranges** — *3 g fiber 1 medium*

5 **Bananas** — *3 g fiber 1 medium*

Most fruits develop from a plant's flower. There are thousands of fruits. Most taste sweet, are low in calories, and have virtually no fat. Fruits deliver a combination of sugars—fructose, glucose, and sucrose—in varying proportions. Fructose is the principal sugar and is the sweetest, although sucrose (common table sugar) is the main sugar in fruits like oranges, melons, and peaches. The calorie content of fruit is kept low by water, which makes up 80–95% of most fruits and gives them their refreshing juiciness.

Ripeness is the key to good fruit. As fruit ripens, its color changes, the vitamin content increases, acidic content decreases, and the starch changes to sugar, giving fruit its mild, sweet flavor and aroma. These changes are caused by enzymes that continue to act on the fruit even after harvesting. Fruit has excellent nutritional value and touches the human spirit, fostering joy and happiness through rich tastes and beautiful colors.

Honorable Mentions

Papaya	6 g fiber in 1 medium
Kiwi	5 g fiber in 2 medium
Blueberries	4 g fiber per 1 cup
Strawberries, sliced	3 g fiber per 1 cup
Guava	3 g fiber in 1 medium
Mango, sliced	3 g fiber per 1 cup
Peach	2 g fiber in 1 medium

Raspberries and Blackberries

FUN FACTS

There are more than 200 species of raspberries grown from the Arctic to the equator. They range in color from yellow to orange to red, purple, and black. Fragrantly sweet and with a subtle, tart overtone, raspberries are a taste sensation. Technically, both the raspberry and blackberry are aggregate fruits—each berry a collection of dozens of tiny fruits. As bramble fruits, raspberries and blackberries are members of the rose family.

abundant vitamin C protects body against oxidative damage

rich source of vitamin B (folate) to guard against heart disease

fiber content of raspberries and blackberries is twice that of strawberries

anthocyanin pigments provide anti-inflammatory and antioxidant benefits

Nutrition Facts

Raspberries and Blackberries
Serving size: 1 cup

Dietary Fiber .... 8 g

Calories	64
Total fat	1 g
Saturated fat	0 g
Trans fat	0 g
Cholesterol	0 mg
Sodium	1 mg
Potassium	186 mg
Total carbohydrate	15 g
Sugars	5 g
Protein	2 g

Pears

FUN FACTS

The pear's delicate flavor and buttery texture have earned it the nickname "butter fruit" in Europe. The Greeks loved pears so much that Homer refers to them in *The Odyssey*. Pears are picked unripe; if left to ripen on the tree, they will have a gritty texture. Pears need to be soft to attain optimum flavor. To speed ripening, place pears in a perforated bag, turning frequently to ensure even ripening. There are more than 5,000 varieties of pears.

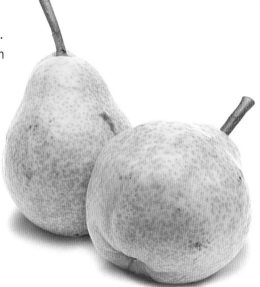

rich source of vitamin A, known to be good for visual acuity, immune function, and healthy skin

high vitamin C content acts as antioxidant and bolsters immune system

contains vitamins and nutrients especially good for health of bones and skin

known as one of the most hypoallergenic foods, those least likely to produce allergic reactions

Nutrition Facts

Pears, raw
Serving size: 1 medium

Dietary Fiber .... 6 g

Calories 103	Trans fat .... 0 g
Total fat .... 0 g	Cholesterol .... 0 mg
Saturated fat .... 0 g	Sodium .... 2 mg
	Potassium .... 212 mg
	Total carbohydrate .... 28 g
	Sugars .... 17 g
	Protein .... 1 g

Apples

FUN FACTS

With about 7500 varieties worldwide, apples are among the most widely consumed fruits on earth, second only to the banana in America. Most of the 2500 varieties grown in the U.S. are hybrids of the apples first brought to America by early colonists who established orchards in Massachusetts and Virginia. Johnny Appleseed was a real person who traveled America in the early 1800s planting apple seeds as he went. (His real name was Johnny Chapman.) Apples float because 25% of their volume is air.

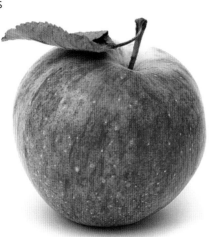

Health Benefits

contains quercetin, a strong antioxidant and anti-inflammatory flavonoid

one of the best foods available to ward off cancer and harmful viruses

high fructose content requires less insulin to digest, forestalling diabetic reactions

fibrous, juicy, and nonsticky, apples are excellent for health of teeth and gums

Nutrition Facts

Apple, raw
Serving size: 1 medium

Dietary Fiber .... 4 g

Calories 95	
Total fat .... 0 g	
Saturated fat .... 0 g	
Trans fat .... 0 g	
Cholesterol .... 0 mg	
Sodium .... 2 mg	
Potassium .... 195 mg	
Total carbohydrate .... 25 g	
Sugars .... 19 g	
Protein .... 0 g	

Oranges

FUN FACTS

One of the most popular fruits in the world, the orange is actually a modified berry with a tough, leathery rind. Rarely found in cooler climates, it was long considered a rare and expensive delicacy. Like all citrus fruits, the orange is acidic, with a pH level of around 2.5 to 3—as strong as vinegar, though not as strong as the lemon. Americans consume most of their oranges in the form of juice. This processing removes most, or all, of the fiber.

Health Benefits

If junk food is the devil, then a sweet orange is as scripture.

—Audrey Foris

high in herperidin, a flavonone thought to lower high blood pressure and cholesterol

rich in flavonoids that inhibit blood clotting and guard against stroke

full of limonoids, compounds that fight cancers of the entire digestive tract

with over 170 phytonutrients, a rich source of daily nutritional requirements

Nutrition Facts

Oranges, raw, all commercial varieties
Serving size: 1 medium

Dietary Fiber .... 3 g

Calories	62
Total fat	0 g
Saturated fat	0 g
Trans fat	0 g
Cholesterol	0 mg
Sodium	0 mg
Potassium	237 mg
Total carbohydrate	15 g
Sugars	12 g
Protein	1 g

Bananas

FUN FACTS

Americans eat more bananas than any other fruit—about 33 pounds per person annually. Although there are more than 500 varieties of bananas, most bananas sold in the U.S. are of the Cavendish variety. Banana trees aren't really trees, botanically speaking, but are classified as the world's largest herb, *Musa sapientium*. Bananas were introduced to the United States in 1876 at its first centennial celebration.

Yeah, I like cars and basketball. But you know what I like more? Bananas.

—Frankie Muniz

rich in vitamin B6, which improves mental function and performance

helps stimulate production of serotonin, elevating mood and alleviating depression

a well-known source of potassium, excellent for lowering blood pressure and plaque in blood vessels

concentrated source of carbohydrates for quick energy and endurance

Nutrition Facts

Bananas, raw
Serving size: 1 medium

Dietary Fiber .... 3 g

Calories	105
Total fat	0 g
Saturated fat	0 g
Trans fat	0 g
Cholesterol	0 mg
Sodium	1 mg
Potassium	422 mg
Total carbohydrate	27 g
Sugars	14 g
Protein	1 g

49

Top 5 Vegetables for Your Diet

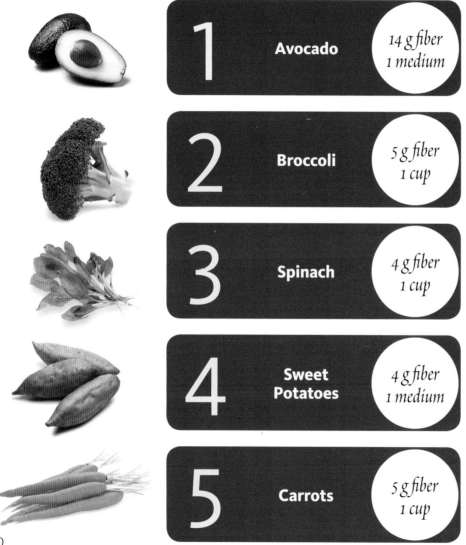

1	**Avocado**	*14 g fiber 1 medium*
2	**Broccoli**	*5 g fiber 1 cup*
3	**Spinach**	*4 g fiber 1 cup*
4	**Sweet Potatoes**	*4 g fiber 1 medium*
5	**Carrots**	*5 g fiber 1 cup*

Vegetables are any flowers, seeds, leaves, buds, stems, tubers, or roots that can be eaten. A diet high in vegetables reduces the risk of chronic diseases including cardiovascular diseases, diabetes, hypertension, stroke, Alzheimer's, digestive disorders, cataracts, and cancer. Vegetables are rich sources of vitamins, minerals, protein, carbohydrates, and fiber and contain a relatively new category of nutrients called phytonutrients or phytochemicals. These are found in all vegetables and have antioxidant, antibacterial, antifungal, antiviral, and anticarcinogenic properties, depending on the plant. The highest concentrations of phytochemicals are found in vegetables with rich colors, intense flavors, and enticing aromas. Brief steaming or rapid boiling in the least possible amount of water results in the smallest loss of nutrients. Notable exceptions are tomatoes and carrots—their nutrient levels are increased with cooking.

Honorable Mentions

Corn	5 g fiber per 1 cup, cooked
Green cabbage	3 g fiber per 1 cup, cooked
Beets, fresh	3 g fiber per 1 cup, cooked
Kale, fresh, chopped	3 g fiber per 1 cup, cooked
Zucchini, sliced	3 g fiber per 1 cup, cooked
Tomatoes, fresh, chopped	2 g fiber per 1 cup
Romaine lettuce, chopped	1 g fiber per 1 cup

Avocado

FUN FACTS

A favorite of the Aztecs, the avocado is native to Central America, with evidence of avocado cultivation in Mexico for thousands of years. Avocados were first cultivated in the United States in the mid-1800s. California produces nearly 90% of the domestic crop.

Avocados will not ripen on the tree. This delay in ripening is a boon to growers, who can leave avocados on the tree for up to 7 months if market conditions aren't favorable when the fruit is first ready to harvest.

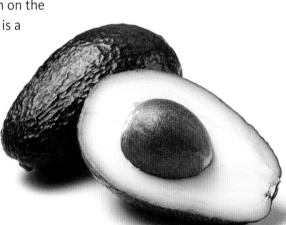

Nutrition Facts

Avocado
Serving size: ½ medium

Dietary Fiber .... 7 g

Calories	161
Total fat	15 g
Saturated fat	2 g
Trans fat	0 g
Cholesterol	0 mg
Sodium	7 mg
Potassium	487 mg
Total carbohydrate	9 g
Sugars	1 g
Protein	2 g

Health Benefits

Avocado is the veritable fruit of paradise.

—David Fairchild

cholesterol-lowering food, second only to olives in monounsaturated (good) fat

contains lots of heart-healthy folate and oleic acid

rich in E, K, and B vitamins, with more potassium than bananas

helps guard against high blood pressure, heart disease, and stroke

Broccoli

FUN FACTS

Broccoli is native to the shores of the Mediterranean. The Italians were the first to cultivate broccoli, and it quickly became a favorite food in ancient Rome. It was introduced to France in the 1500s, and then to England in the mid-18th century. Broccoli arrived in America during colonial times. George Washington and Thomas Jefferson both grew it in their kitchen gardens. California and Arizona produce 99% of the U.S. broccoli crop.

supplies vitamin C, necessary for building healthy blood vessels and cartilage

prevents anemia by enhancing the absorption of iron from other foods

assists in making thyroxin, which regulates the metabolic rate

a gold mine of potent cancer-fighting chemicals such as beta carotene

Nutrition Facts

Broccoli
Serving size: 1 cup, cooked, without salt

Dietary Fiber .... 5 g

Calories 55	Trans fat .... 0 g
Total fat .... 1 g	Cholesterol .... 0 mg
Saturated fat .... 0 g	Sodium .... 64 mg
	Potassium .... 457 mg
	Total carbohydrate .... 11 g
	Sugars .... 2 g
	Protein .... 4 g

Spinach

Spinach was the favorite vegetable of Catherine de Medici during the Renaissance. When she left Florence, Italy, to marry the king of France, she brought along her own cooks so they could prepare spinach in the ways she preferred. Since that time, dishes prepared on a bed of spinach are referred to as "à la Florentine." The United States and the Netherlands are the largest producers of spinach. Varieties include baby spoon, flat or smooth leaf, red, savoy, and semi savoy.

Health Benefits

I'm strong to the finish
'cause I eats me spinach.

—Popeye

calorie for calorie, provides more nutrients than any other food

high in lutein, a carotenoid that protects against macular degeneration and cataracts

an excellent source of iron, especially important for women

reduces symptoms of asthma, osteoarthritis, osteoporosis, and rheumatoid arthritis

Nutrition Facts

Spinach
Serving size: 1 cup fresh, cooked

Dietary Fiber .... 4 g

Calories	41
Total fat	0 g
Saturated fat	0 g
Trans fat	0 g
Cholesterol	0 mg
Sodium	126 mg
Potassium	839 mg
Total carbohydrate	7 g
Sugars	1 g
Protein	5 g

Sweet Potatoes

FUN FACTS

Sweet potatoes aren't related to white potatoes at all, but are in the morning glory family. One of the oldest known vegetables, the sweet potato is native to the New World and has been found in pre-Incan ruins in Peru. Columbus brought sweet potatoes to Europe after his first voyage in 1492. They were a popular aphrodisiac in Shakespeare's day. North Carolina is the leading sweet potato producer in the U.S., followed by California, Louisiana, and Mississippi.

Health Benefits

ranked by food scientists as the most nutritious of all vegetables

excellent source of minerals such as potassium, iron, manganese, and copper

a perfect blend of everything needed for long-lasting energy

abundant in the "cancer-fighting ninjas"—quercetin and chlorogenic acid

Nutrition Facts

Sweet Potatoes
Serving size: 1 medium, baked in skin, without salt

Dietary Fiber .... 4 g

Calories	103
Total fat	0 g
Saturated fat	0 g
Trans fat	0 g
Cholesterol	0 mg
Sodium	41 mg
Potassium	542 mg
Total carbohydrate	24 g
Sugars	7 g
Protein	2 g

Carrots

FUN FACTS

Carrots were esteemed for their medicinal value prior to the time of Christ. Settlers arriving in Virginia were the first to bring carrot seeds to America. Originally, purple carrots came from the region now known as Afghanistan 5000 years ago. Beta III carrots have 5 times the beta carotene of regular carrots. Maroon carrots are sweeter than regular carrots and have a porous texture like celery or apples. Look for leafy tops that are crisp and green, an indication of freshness.

Health Benefits

Did you ever stop to taste a carrot? Not just eat it, but taste it? You can't taste the beauty and energy of the earth in a Twinkie.

—Astrid Alauda

supplies calcium pectate, a soluble fiber that helps remove LDL (bad) cholesterol from the body

high in beta carotene, from which the body makes vitamin A

very low in calories, with virtually no fat—a superlative diet food

antioxidant and anti-cancer properties in beta carotene

Nutrition Facts

Carrots
Serving size: ½ cup sliced, cooked, without salt

Dietary Fiber .... 2 g

Calories	27
Total fat	0 g
Saturated fat	0 g
Trans fat	0 g
Cholesterol	0 mg
Sodium	45 mg
Potassium	183 mg
Total carbohydrate	6 g
Sugars	3 g
Protein	1 g

Top 5 Beans for Your Diet

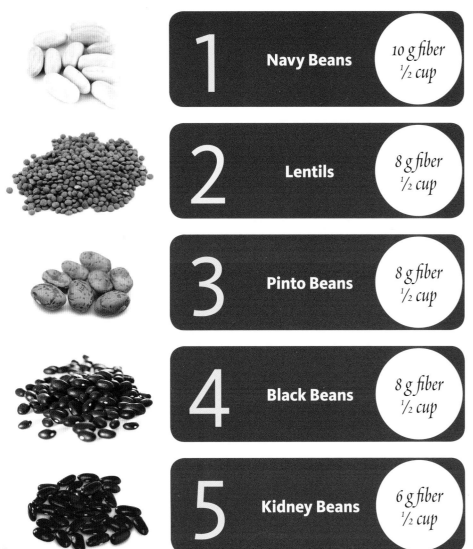

1 **Navy Beans** — 10 g fiber ½ cup

2 **Lentils** — 8 g fiber ½ cup

3 **Pinto Beans** — 8 g fiber ½ cup

4 **Black Beans** — 8 g fiber ½ cup

5 **Kidney Beans** — 6 g fiber ½ cup

Beans are super-foods because of their nutritional content, which includes protein, fiber, iron, manganese, magnesium, folate, antioxidants, and phytochemicals. In the 1600s, Native Americans taught European settlers how to plant beans and corn together so that the bean vines would climb the cornstalks for support. Some people avoid beans because they're concerned about intestinal gas side effects. The gas is caused by intestinal bacteria breaking down the natural sugars found in beans. This sugar is water soluble and is on the surface of the bean, so if you soak dry beans overnight and then drain off the water before cooking them in fresh water, the gas problems will go away. Beans are an excellent source of protein. One cup has twice as much protein as a cup of milk, equal to a 2-ounce serving of beef or fish. Beans are unsurpassed in fiber content.

Honorable Mentions

Lima beans, large	7 g fiber per ½ cup, cooked
Garbanzo beans	6 g fiber per ½ cup, cooked
Black-eyed peas	6 g fiber per ½ cup, cooked
Green peas	4 g fiber per ½ cup, cooked
Green beans	2 g fiber per ½ cup, cooked

Navy Beans

FUN FACTS

Navy beans got their name during the years when Theodore Roosevelt was Assistant Secretary of the Navy. They were a staple food of the U.S. Navy during most of the 20th century. Small, dense and smooth, creamy white and mild in flavor, these are the beans used for the famous Boston and English baked beans. With nearly 150,000 acres committed to the effort, Michigan leads the nation in the production of navy beans.

Health Benefits

soluble fiber helps control cholesterol and blood sugar and prevents diabetes

insoluble fiber aids in preventing constipation by stimulating the digestive tract

bean protein is kinder to the body, especially the kidneys, than meat protein

good source of complex carbohydrates, sustaining energy and satiety for hours

Nutrition Facts

Navy Beans
Serving size: ½ cup, cooked, without salt

Dietary Fiber .... 10 g

Calories	127
Total fat	1 g
Saturated fat	0 g
Trans fat	0 g
Cholesterol	0 mg
Sodium	0 mg
Potassium	354 mg
Total carbohydrate	24 g
Sugars	0 g
Protein	7 g

Lentils

FUN FACTS

Named for their distinctive lens shape, lentils are mentioned four times in the Bible, most famously as the ingredient in the soup for which Esau sold his inheritance to his younger brother, Jacob. In colors ranging from yellow to orange to red, green, brown, and black, lentils are sold whole or split, with or without the skins. Lentils have a high drought tolerance, so they can be grown in semi-arid regions—in the U.S., the Palouse Region of eastern Washington and the Idaho Panhandle.

Health Benefits

Current thinking is that the lentil is one of nature's most perfect foods.

—Jon Carroll

rich in folate and copper, both of which contribute to red blood cell production

protein and fiber content satisfy for hours after eating, helping control appetite

saponins and inositol hexaphosphate reduce risk of cancer

as seeds, chock-full of the energy needed for the early growth of the new plant

Nutrition Facts

Lentils
Serving size: ½ cup, cooked, without salt

Dietary Fiber .... 8 g

Calories	115
Total fat	0 g
Saturated fat	0 g
Trans fat	0 g
Cholesterol	0 mg
Sodium	2 mg
Potassium	365 mg
Total Carbohydrate	20 g
Sugars	2 g
Protein	9 g

Pinto Beans

FUN FACTS

Pinto means "painted," and dry pinto beans have a mottled surface that appears painted. When cooked, this mottling disappears and the beans adopt a uniform color. They are the most commonly consumed bean in America, with the average American consuming 4 pounds (dry weight) per year. Dove Creek, Colorado, is the "pinto bean capital of the world."

high in folic acid, which helps reduce inflammation in artery walls

contains molybdenum, which helps detoxify sulfite preservatives used in packaged foods

rich in thiamine (vitamin B1), essential for good memory function

high in iron, essential for production of oxygen-transporting hemoglobin

Nutrition Facts

Pinto Beans
Serving size: ½ cup, cooked, without salt

Dietary Fiber .... 8 g

Calories	122
Total fat	1 g
Saturated fat	0 g
Trans fat	0 g
Cholesterol	0 mg
Sodium	1 mg
Potassium	373 mg
Total Carbohydrate	22g
Sugars	0 g
Protein	8 g

59

Black Beans

FUN FACTS

Black beans came to Europe when Spanish conquistadors returned from their voyages to the New World. Spanish and Portuguese traders carried them into Africa and Asia. Black beans have a rich, smoky flavor that has been compared to mushrooms; they have a velvety texture, yet hold their shape well during cooking. They are an important source of protein in the cuisines of Mexico, Brazil, Cuba, Guatemala, and the Dominican Republic.

Health Benefits

unlike canned vegetables, canned beans retain all nutritional value

high in saponins that lower cholesterol levels by preventing reabsorption into the bloodstream

as seeds, beans are nutrient reservoirs—energy, protein, vitamin, and mineral accumulators

studies of adults over 70 indicate that bean consumption increases longevity

Nutrition Facts

Black Beans
Serving size: ½ cup, cooked, without salt

Dietary Fiber .... 8 g

Calories	114
Total fat	0 g
Saturated fat	0 g
Trans fat	0 g
Sodium	1 mg
Potassium	305 mg
Total carbohydrate	20 g
Protein	8 g

Kidney Beans

FUN FACTS

Originating in Peru, kidney beans were carried by native traders into Central America where they were discovered by the Spanish monks who accompanied the European explorers. Kidney beans are part of Louisiana's famous red beans and rice. These regal red, kidney-shaped beans must be boiled for at least 10 minutes to destroy their natural phytohemagglutinin, and then cooked until tender. Failure to boil these beans could lead to unpleasant gastric symptoms. (Canned beans have been fully boiled.)

Health Benefits

Red beans and ricely yours.

—Louis Armstrong

high soluble fiber content helps reduce cholesterol and stabilize blood sugar

magnesium and potassium content good for lowering blood pressure

rich in manganese and copper, helping protect against cancer and vascular disease

with little fat and no cholesterol, an excellent substitute for meat protein

Nutrition Facts

Kidney Beans
Serving size: ½ cup, cooked, without salt

Dietary Fiber .... 6 g

Calories 112	Trans fat .... 0 g
Total fat .... 0 g	Cholesterol .... 0 mg
Saturated fat .... 0 g	Sodium .... 1 mg
	Potassium .... 358 mg
	Total carbohydrate .... 20 g
	Sugars .... 0 g
	Protein .... 8 g

Top 5 Nuts & Seeds for Your Diet

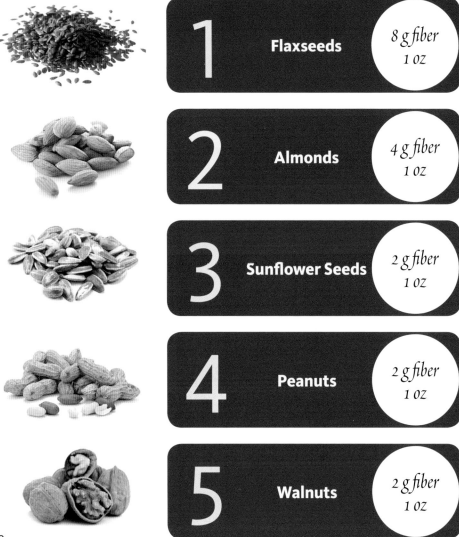

1 Flaxseeds — *8 g fiber* 1 oz

2 Almonds — *4 g fiber* 1 oz

3 Sunflower Seeds — *2 g fiber* 1 oz

4 Peanuts — *2 g fiber* 1 oz

5 Walnuts — *2 g fiber* 1 oz

Americans tend to think of nuts as snack foods, but they're much more nourishing than that. Seeds and nuts deserve a place in our daily meals. Seeds and nuts grow all over the world and are very versatile in cooking. Their reputation has been transformed in recent years from high-fat villains to nutritional heroes. These fat-rich delights, once considered a no-no when trying to lose weight, have now been recognized as weight loss aids when eaten in moderation and in place of other fatty foods. The majority of their fat is the healthy unsaturated kind, with well-known cholesterol-lowering, heart-healthy benefits. Seeds and nuts offer vitamin E, B1, B2, B6, panothenic acid, and folate. They also provide calcium, iron, magnesium, and phosphorus. They're rich in the trace minerals zinc, manganese, copper, and selenium, all of which help defend our bodies against oxidative damage.

Honorable Mentions

Chia seeds	11 g fiber in 1 oz
Pecans	3 g fiber in 1 oz
Hazelnuts (filberts)	3 g fiber in 1 oz
Brazil nuts	2 g fiber in 1 oz
Pumpkin seeds	1 g fiber in 1 oz

Flaxseeds

Flax fiber is the source of linen, and other parts of the plant are used to make fabric, dye, paper, medicines, fishing nets, and soap. Charlemagne made flax popular in European culture. Impressed with its versatility, he passed laws requiring its cultivation and consumption. Canada is currently the leading producer of flaxseeds in the world, followed by China, India, and the United States. Nearly 100% of the U.S. crop is raised in North Dakota, South Dakota, and Minnesota.

Health Benefits

reduces attention deficit hyperactivity disorder (ADHD) by protecting neurons

rich source of omega-3 fat, which provides protection from cognitive decline and depression

decreases severity of autoimmune diseases and promotes bone health

omega-3 fat reduces the risk of dry eye syndrome

Nutrition Facts

Flaxseeds
Serving size: 2 Tbsp

Dietary Fiber .... 6 g

Calories 110	Trans fat .... 0 g
Total fat .... 9 g	Cholesterol .... 0 mg
Saturated fat .... 1 g	Sodium .... 6 mg
	Potassium .... 167 mg
	Total Carbohydrate .... 6 g
	Sugars .... 0 g
	Protein .... 4 g

Almonds

FUN FACTS

The almond is actually the seed of the fruit of the almond tree and is related to the other stone fruits like peaches, apricots, and plums. Almonds are mentioned 10 times in the Bible, beginning in the book of Genesis. California is the only state that produces almonds. With its soft texture, mild flavor, and light color, the almond can be eaten raw or toasted. When pressed, it yields a nutritious, delicately flavored almond milk, a delightful alternative to cow's milk.

Health Benefits

good source of vitamin B2 (riboflavin), niacin, folate, potassium, other minerals

calcium content good for bones, muscles, nerve function, blood pressure, immune defenses

highest of all nuts in fiber content— 4 grams per ounce

lowers risk of diabetes and heart disease by moderating insulin spikes

Nutrition Facts

Almonds
Serving size: 1 oz (23)

Dietary Fiber .... 4 g

Calories 163	Trans fat .... 0 g
Total fat .... 14 g	Cholesterol .... 0 mg
Saturated fat .... 1 g	Sodium .... 0 mg
	Potassium .... 200 mg
	Total carbohydrate .... 6 g
	Sugars .... 1 g
	Protein .... 6 g

Sunflower Seeds

Sunflower seeds come from the familiar, large, daisy-like flower of the sunflower plant, which can grow as tall as 10 feet. Native Americans used the seeds as a snack, pounded them into meal, cooked them as a mash, and used them to make bread. Around 1500, Spanish explorers took the plants to Europe. By the 18th century, it was discovered that the seeds were valuable for their oil. The Russians remain the world's top producer of the seeds to this day.

Health Benefits

outstanding source of E, the antioxidant vitamin

alleviate severity and frequency of hot flashes in menopausal women

phytosterol content helps lower blood cholesterol levels

reduce risk of colon cancer

Nutrition Facts

Sunflower seeds, hulled

Serving size: ¼ cup

Dietary Fiber .... 3 g

Calories	204
Total fat	18 g
Saturated fat	2 g
Trans fat	0 g
Cholesterol	0 mg
Sodium	3 mg
Potassium	226 mg
Total Carbohydrate	7 g
Sugars	1 g
Protein	7 g

Peanuts

FUN FACTS

One of the most popular nuts in the United States, peanuts are not true nuts but legumes, like peas and beans. In 1870, P.T. Barnum began offering roasted peanuts in his circus as a snack food. Soon they began showing up in ballparks and movie theaters. Botanist George Washington Carver researched peanuts at Tuskegee Institute in Alabama, where he developed hundreds of uses for the peanut, including cosmetics, dyes, paints, plastics, gasoline, and nitroglycerin.

Health Benefits

rich source of cholesterol-lowering plant sterols

good source of niacin, which lowers risk of Alzheimer's disease

high monounsaturated fat—good for reducing body fat

significant resveratrol content cuts risk of cardiovascular disease

Nutrition Facts

Peanuts, all types, dry-roasted

Serving size: 1 oz (28)

Dietary Fiber .... 2 g

Calories 166	
Total fat .... 14 g	
Saturated fat .... 2 g	
Trans fat .... 0 g	
Cholesterol .... 0 mg	
Sodium .... 2 mg	
Potassium .... 187 mg	
Total carbohydrate .... 6 g	
Sugars .... 1 g	
Protein .... 7 g	

Walnuts

FUN FACTS

In the 18th century, Franciscan monks planted walnuts in California, where the mild climate and fertile soil provided ideal growing conditions. California now provides 99% of the United States' and 67% of the world's supply of walnuts. The walnut's botanical name, *Juglans regia*, comes from the Romans and means "the royal acorn of Jupiter." The Afghani word for walnut is *charmarghz* or "four brains" because of the unique shape of the walnut kernel. Walnut trees can live for 250 years.

Health Benefits

high levels of amino acid L-arginine help control hypertension

ellagic acid strengthens the immune system and helps prevent breast and prostate cancer

omega-3 fatty acids protect against rheumatoid arthritis, lupus, eczema, and psoriasis

with 16 polyphenols, walnuts have the highest antioxidant content of the tree nuts

Nutrition Facts

Walnuts, English
Serving size: 1 oz (14 halves)

Dietary Fiber .... 2 g

Calories 185	
Total fat .... 18 g	
Saturated fat .... 2 g	
Trans fat .... 0 g	
Cholesterol .... 0 mg	
Sodium .... 1 mg	
Potassium .... 125 mg	
Total carbohydrate .... 4 g	
Sugars .... 1 g	
Protein .... 4 g	

Top 5 Grains for Your Diet

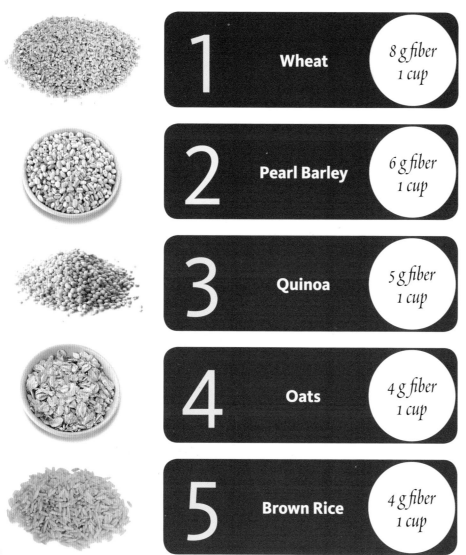

1 **Wheat** — *8 g fiber 1 cup*

2 **Pearl Barley** — *6 g fiber 1 cup*

3 **Quinoa** — *5 g fiber 1 cup*

4 **Oats** — *4 g fiber 1 cup*

5 **Brown Rice** — *4 g fiber 1 cup*

Grains are the seed-like fruit produced by grasses such as wheat, oats, barley, corn, rice, rye, amaranth, triticale, quinoa, millet, and sorghum. Whole grains include all parts of the grain: the bran (containing most of the grain's fiber), endosperm (kernel containing the grain's starch and protein), and the germ (which forms new plants and contains antioxidants, vitamins B and E, and trace minerals). "Enriched" means a grain has been processed to remove the nutritious bran and germ, leaving behind only the starchy endosperm, which is made into white flour. Small amounts of vitamins and minerals are then added back into the flour, thus "enriching" it. Look at the ingredient list. Make sure it says "whole" before the name of the grain. Terms such as enriched, bleached, unbleached, stone ground, hearty grain, multi-grain, cracked, milled, or "100%" before the name of the grain are often marketing ploys. These products are not necessarily whole grain and will be deficient in nutrition and fiber.

Honorable Mentions

Rye flakes	5 g fiber per 1 cup, cooked
Buckwheat groats	5 g fiber per 1 cup, cooked
Whole-grain cornmeal	3 g fiber per 1 cup, cooked
Wild rice	3 g fiber per 1 cup, cooked
Millet	2 g fiber per 1 cup, cooked

Wheat

FUN FACTS

Wheat nourishes more of the world's people than any other grain. Columbus brought it to the West in the late 15th century. Today the U.S. is among the top wheat-growing nations of the world. Winter wheat is planted in autumn and harvested in the spring. Spring wheat is planted in the spring, harvested in late summer. Wheat grains have three layers: bran, endosperm, and germ. Vitamins, minerals, and phytochemicals reside mainly in the bran and germ. Kamut and spelt, also called farro, are two ancient strains of wheat sold mostly in in health food stores.

Health Benefits

bran and germ layers rich in vitamins, minerals, and phytochemicals

whole-grain wheat provides health benefits absent from refined, white flour

bran and germ are rich in disease-fighting flavonoids, lignans, saponins, and phytosterols

whole-grain wheat protects against weight gain and aids in weight loss

Nutrition Facts

Wheat Bulgur
Serving size: 1 cup, cooked, without salt

Dietary Fiber .... 8 g

Calories 151	Trans fat .... 0 g
Total fat .... 0 g	Cholesterol .... 0 mg
Saturated fat .... 0 g	Sodium .... 9 mg
	Potassium .... 124 mg
	Total Carbohydrate .... 34 g
	Sugars .... 0 g
	Protein .... 6 g

Pearl Barley

FUN FACTS

References to barley are found in Egyptian writings more than 5000 years old. Barley has a chewy, pasta-like consistency and is covered with a tough, inedible hull that must be removed by a mechanical sanding process called "pearling." The more the barley is pearled, the lighter it will be in color.
Much of the barley grown in the U.S. is soaked until it sprouts and then used to make beer, but barley is much more nutritious as a cereal added to other foods.

high in manganese, a co-factor for more than 300 important enzymes

rich in selenium, an essential component of thyroid hormone metabolism

high in phosphorus, required for bone and tooth formation

good source of copper, required for critical enzymes to function properly

Nutrition Facts

Barley, pearl
Serving size: 1 cup, cooked, without salt

Dietary Fiber .... 6 g

Calories 193	Trans fat .... 0 g
Total fat ....1 g	Cholesterol.................................... 0 mg
Saturated fat .... 0 g	Sodium .... 5 mg
	Potassium .... 146 mg
	Total carbohydrate .... 44 g
	Sugars .... 0 g
	Protein .... 4 g

Quinoa

FUN FACTS

Quinoa (KEEN-wah) is not a true grain, but the seed of a leafy vegetable. The Incas considered it sacred, calling it the *chisaya mama* or "mother of all grains," and the emperor sowed the first seeds of each season using golden implements. In the 1980s, two Americans, learning of its nutritional benefits, began cultivating it in Colorado. Quinoa has a low gluten content, making it an ideal grain for those who are gluten intolerant.

Health Benefits

rich in high-quality protein, even more than oats

contains high levels of all 9 essential amino acids, especially lysine

good source of iron to protect against anemia, especially important for women

high riboflavin content cuts frequency of migraine occurrence

Nutrition Facts

Quinoa
Serving size: 1 cup, cooked, without salt

Dietary Fiber .... 5 g

Calories	222
Total fat	4 g
Saturated fat	0 g
Trans fat	0 g
Cholesterol	0 mg
Sodium	13 mg
Potassium	318 mg
Total carbohydrate	39 g
Sugars	2 g
Protein	8 g

Oats

FUN FACTS

"Oats are only fit to be fed to horses and Scotsmen" is a traditional saying in England. To which the Scottish reply is, "and England has the finest horses, and Scotland the finest men." Oats offer powerful nutrition. Oat extract soothes the skin, which is why it's the basis of the Aveeno products. (*Avena* is the genus to which oats belong.) Oats prefer the cool, wet summers of Northwest Europe. They can even be grown in Iceland.

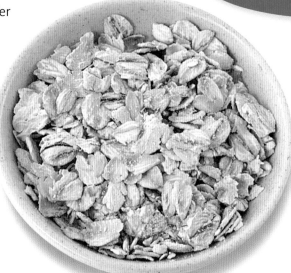

Health Benefits

We load up on oat bran in the morning so we'll live forever. Then we spend the rest of the day living like there's no tomorrow.

—Lee Iacocca

oats supply 50% more protein than wheat, 100% more than rice

best source of cholesterol-lowering beta-glucan, which also regulates blood sugar

slow-digesting starches stabilize blood sugar levels

well-known ability to lower cholesterol and maintain healthy blood flow

Nutrition Facts

Oatmeal
Serving size: 1 cup, cooked, without salt

Dietary Fiber .... 4 g

Calories 166	
Total fat .... 4 g	
Saturated fat .... 1 g	
Trans fat .... 0 g	
Cholesterol .... 0 mg	
Sodium .... 9 mg	
Potassium .... 164 mg	
Total carbohydrate .... 28 g	
Sugars .... 1 g	
Protein .... 6 g	

Brown Rice

Rice is grown on every continent except Antarctica and is the staple food for half the world's population. The milling and polishing that converts brown rice into white rice destroys 67% of the vitamin B3, 80% of the vitamin B1, 90% of the vitamin B6, 50% of the manganese, 50% of the phosphorus, 60% of the iron, and 100% of the dietary fiber and essential fatty acids. Brown rice is much healthier than white rice. It has a mild nutty flavor.

Health Benefits

low in calories and fat, brown rice is virtually sodium-free

contains oryzanol, a powerful antioxidant, in its outer layers

one cup of brown rice provides 88% of daily manganese for a healthy nervous system

guards against cancer, heart disease, dementia, and aging

Nutrition Facts

Rice, brown, long-grain
Serving size: 1 cup, cooked, without salt

Dietary Fiber .... 4 g

Calories	216
Total fat	2 g
Saturated fat	0 g
Trans fat	0 g
Cholesterol	0 mg
Sodium	10 mg
Potassium	84 mg
Carbohydrate	45 g
Sugars	1 g
Protein	5 g

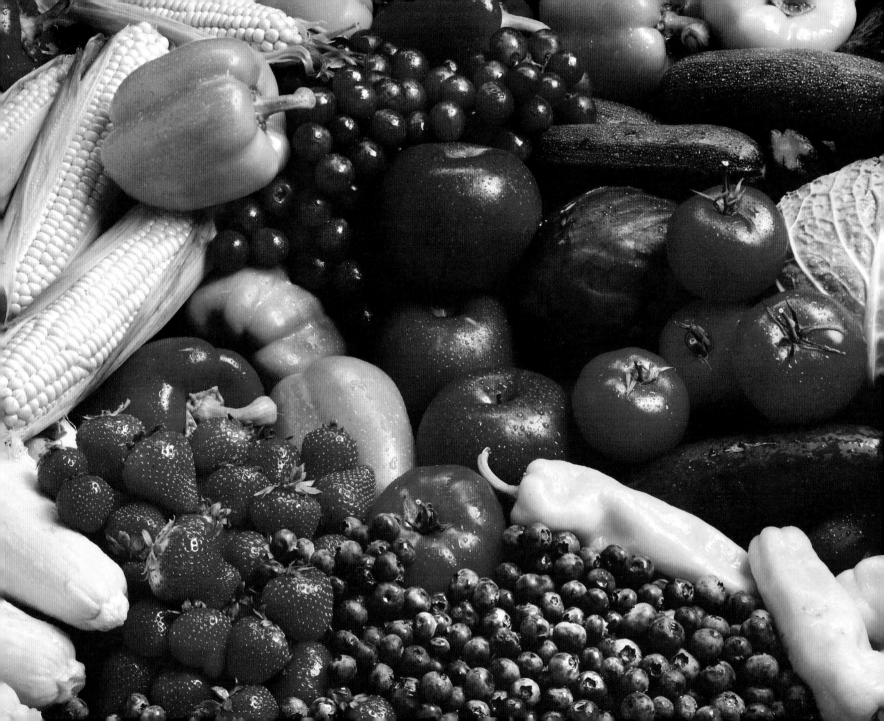

CHAPTER SIX

Adding Fiber to Foods You Already Eat

They always say time changes things, but you actually have to change them yourself.

—Andy Warhol
The Philosophy of Andy Warhol

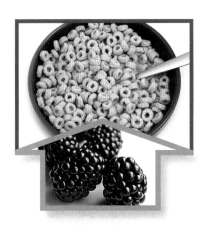

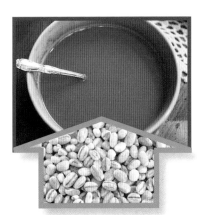

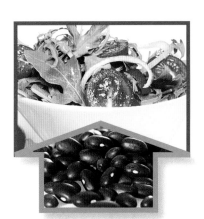

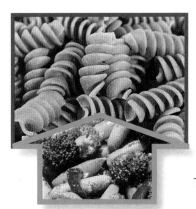

The Fiber Power Up

Most Americans eat less than 10 grams of fiber per day. Not knowing any better, they choose high-calorie, processed foods with most of the fiber removed. Consequently, it takes a lot more of these foods to satisfy the hunger.

Bottom line: processed foods are making us fat.

These next few pages will open your eyes to the great-tasting fiber foods readily available and show you how to "power-up" your preferred food choices.

On the left are pictures of commonly eaten foods. The pictures on the right are power-up versions of the same food. We're betting when you see the Power Ups you will say "Wow!, it really is easy to eat more fiber"—and, "I can do that!"

Fiber Power Ups are simple. Start using this big idea and you will see results. You'll eat a full plate of great-tasting food, keep that "full" feeling longer, and consequently consume fewer calories without ever knowing it.

A few weeks from now you'll step onto the scales, look down at the number, and laugh.

A few short weeks later, people will start looking at you differently.

In a good way.

A very good way.

Fiber Face-Off—Head to Head

VS

THE REGULAR

THE POWER UPS

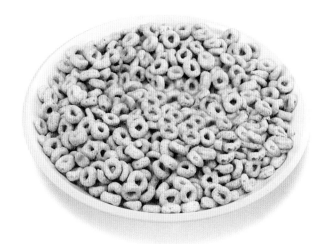

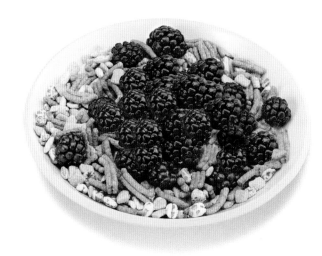

Examples	Serving Amount	Fiber Grams
THE REGULAR		
Cheerios MultiGrain	1 cup	3
Milk	1 cup	0
TOTAL		**3**

Examples	Serving Amount	Fiber Grams
FIBER POWER UP		
Kashi GoLean	1 cup	10
Blackberries	1 cup	8
Milk	1 cup	0
TOTAL		**18**

Fiber Face-Off—Head to Head

VS

FAST FOOD

THE POWER UPS

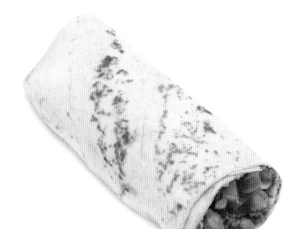

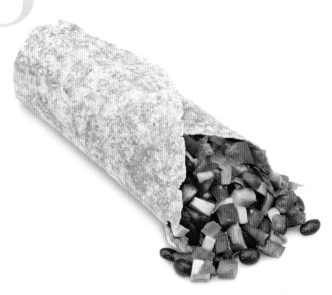

Examples	Serving Amount	Fiber Grams
THE REGULAR		
Taco Bell Fresco Bean Burrito	1	9
TOTAL		**9**

Examples	Serving Amount	Fiber Grams
FIBER POWER UP		
La Tortilla Factory Tortilla Soft Wrap	1	12
Black beans, cooked	½ cup	8
Lettuce, chopped	1 cup	1
Tomato, chopped	½ cup	1
Onion, chopped	2 Tbsp	0
Salsa	¼ cup	1
Avocado	¼ cup	4
TOTAL		**27**

Fiber Face-Off—Head to Head

VS

THE REGULAR

THE POWER UPS

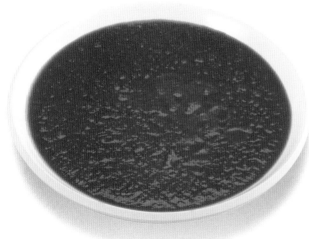

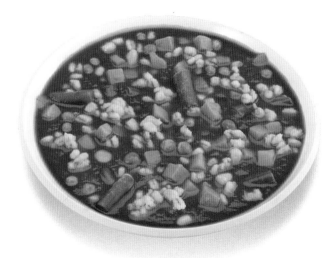

Examples	Serving Amount	Fiber Grams
THE REGULAR		
Cream of tomato soup	1 cup	2
TOTAL		**2**

Examples	Serving Amount	Fiber Grams
FIBER POWER UP		
Cream of tomato soup	1 cup	2
Barley, cooked	½ cup	3
Frozen or fresh vegetables, cooked	½ cup	4
TOTAL		**9**

Fiber Face-Off—Head to Head

VS

THE REGULAR

THE POWER UPS

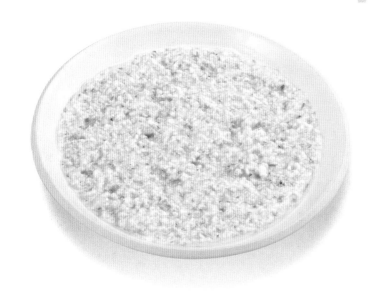

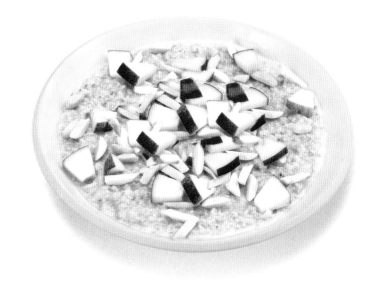

Examples	Serving Amount	Fiber Grams
THE REGULAR		
Oatmeal, cooked	1 cup	4
Milk	½ cup	0
Sugar	1 tsp	0
TOTAL		**4**

Examples	Serving Amount	Fiber Grams
FIBER POWER UP		
Oatmeal, cooked	1 cup	4
Milk	½ cup	0
Apple, chopped	1 medium	4
Slivered almonds	1 oz.	4
TOTAL		**12**

Fiber Face-Off—Head to Head

VS

THE REGULAR

THE POWER UPS

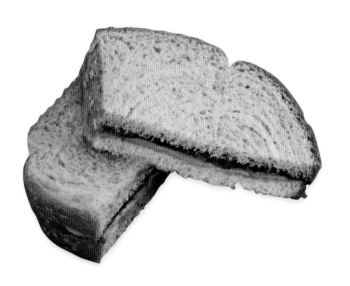

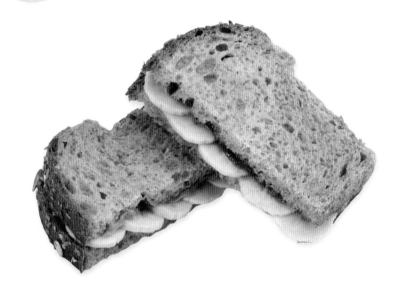

Examples	Serving Amount	Fiber Grams
THE REGULAR		
Wheat bread (not whole wheat)	2 slices	0
Smooth peanut butter	2 Tbsp	2
Jelly	1 tsp	0
TOTAL		**2**

Examples	Serving Amount	Fiber Grams
FIBER POWER UP		
Orowheat Double Fiber whole grain bread	2 slices	12
Crunchy peanut butter	2 tablespoons	3
Banana, sliced	1 medium	3
TOTAL		**18**

Fiber Face-Off—Head to Head

VS

THE REGULAR

THE POWER UPS

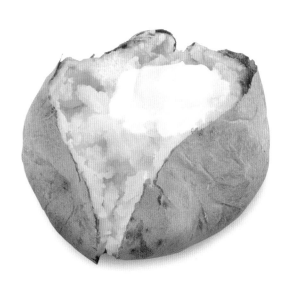

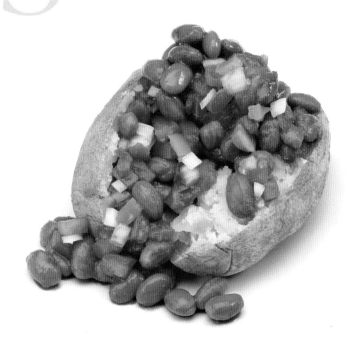

Examples	Serving Amount	Fiber Grams
THE REGULAR		
Baked potato, with skin	1 medium	4
Sour cream	1 Tbsp	0
Butter	1 Tbsp	0
TOTAL		**4**

Examples	Serving Amount	Fiber Grams
FIBER POWER UP		
Baked potato, with skin	1 medium	4
Chili beans	1 cup	12
Salsa	¼ cup	1
TOTAL		**17**

The Fiber Wheel—Quick & Easy Recipes

Each Fiber Wheel is a commonly eaten dish surrounded by many ingredients you might consider adding to it. Hopefully, you'll notice some high-fiber additions to meals you already enjoy and say, "Hey! That would taste good!"—and, "That looks easy, I can do that!"

Remember:

1. Weight loss is all about calorie reduction. For faster weight loss, stick to our recommended serving sizes for nuts, avocados, olives, and oils.
2. Fiber foods fill you up and contain fewer calories.
3. Eat more fiber and you'll have less room for calorie-concentrated foods.
4. We're absolutely NOT saying, "Don't eat this. Don't eat that." Those diets fail. We want you to have a sustainable way of reduced-calorie dining that doesn't feel restrictive to you. Just use the Fiber Wheel and the information on the opposing left-hand page to create your own meal that suits your taste and time.
5. Eat as many vegetables, beans, whole grains, and fruits as you want. Everything else will take care of itself.
6. Yes, it really is that simple.
7. Meat and dairy? No problem. Just eat your fiber first, then drink some water. (And leaving food on your plate is a *good* thing. Meat and dairy have lots of calories.)

For more recipes, go to
www.fullplatediet.org/recipes

> I find a recipe is only a theme, which an intelligent cook can play each time with a variation.
>
> —Madame Jehane Benoit

FUN FACTS

One-third of all recipes for salad in 1930 were for Jell-O salads. Coleslaw got its name from the Dutch *kool sla*—"cabbage salad." Oscar Tschirky created the Waldorf salad in 1893 for the pre-opening of the Waldorf Astoria Hotel in New York. Bob Cobb of The Brown Derby restaurant in L.A. created the Cobb salad as a way to use up leftovers. Lots of people claim to have invented the Caesar salad, but the honor belongs to Caesar Cardini. When his restaurant ran low on food in 1924, he used whole romaine leaves to "fill" the plate—and told patrons to eat the leaves with their fingers so they'd focus on the novelty and not the salad.

STUART'S FAVE

When I entertain I like to use all the spokes of the Salad Fiber Wheel. I display bowls of greens, beans, nuts, tortilla chips, brown rice, salsa, lemon wedges, and assorted peppers. My guests pile their plates high with whatever suits their fancy to create a taco salad. The best part is that no recipes are needed.

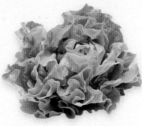

Getting Started

Here are 6 different salads that can be made using the ingredients listed on the opposite page:

* Green Salad—fresh spinach, sliced strawberries, and almonds
* Multi-Bean Salad—garbanzos, kidney beans, green beans, chopped red pepper, marinated in Italian dressing
* Tropical Coleslaw—shredded cabbage and carrots, mandarin oranges, lemon yogurt, chopped walnuts
* Taco Salad—romaine, bell peppers, black beans, tortilla chips, topped with salsa
* Pasta Salad—whole-wheat pasta shells, tomatoes, onions, with Italian dressing
* Tabouli—bulgur wheat (soaked in double amount of boiling water), chopped cucumber, tomatoes, and onions; season to taste with lemon juice, a bit of olive oil, and if you are lucky enough to have them, garnish with fresh mint and parsley. These fresh herbs grow easily in pots on a sunny windowsill or patio.

Good Foods from Your Store

Eden Organic Great Northern Beans	½ cup, cooked	8 g
Guiltless Gourmet Natural Tortilla Chips	1 oz (18 chips)	2 g

Dressings

Newman's Own Lighten Up Italian Dressing	2 Tbsp	0 g
Ortega Salsa Verde	¼ cup	0 g

Just a Little Caution

Dressings, unless they are fat-free, can add lots of calories to a salad, so serve the salad dressing on the side. Be especially careful of the creamy ones—like Ranch dressing.

Salad Fiber Wheel

Greens
(Serving size = 2 cups)
Romaine Lettuce (2 g), Fresh Spinach (2 g),
Cabbage (shredded) (4 g), Spring Mix (2 g)

Fruit
(Serving size = ½ cup, chopped)
Mandarin Oranges (canned, drained) (1 g),
Kiwi (3 g), Berries (3 g), Grapes (0 g)

Vegetables
(Serving size = ½ cup, sliced)
Tomatoes (1 g), Cucumber (0 g),
Onion (1 g), Sweet Green Peppers (1 g)

Whole Grains
(Serving size = 1 cup, cooked)
Spiral Pasta (6 g), Tortilla Chips (1 oz) (3 g),
Brown Rice (4 g), Bulgur Wheat (8 g)

Nuts
(Serving size = 2 Tbsp)
Almonds (sliced) (1 g), Pecans (halved) (1 g),
Sunflower Seeds (2 g), Walnuts (chopped) (1 g)

Meats/Dairy
(Serving size = 3 oz)
Cheese (1 oz) (0 g), Chicken (0 g),
Salmon (0 g), Lean Beef (0 g)

Beans/Legumes
(Serving size = ½ cup, cooked)
Garbanzos (6 g), Kidney Beans (6 g),
Black Beans (8 g), Green Beans (2 g)

Dressings
(Serving size = 2 Tbsp)
Salsa (0 g), Italian (0 g),
Yogurt (0 g), Lemon Juice (0 g)

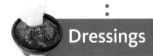
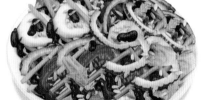

FUN FACTS

Pancakes—cakes cooked in a pan—are as old as the Bible, and waffles were sold outside medieval churches during religious celebrations. In 1561, competition between waffle sellers became so heated that King Charles IX of France made a law requiring them to maintain a distance of at least *deux toises* (6 ft) from one another. Thomas Jefferson brought a waffle iron home from France in 1789. "We hold these truths to be self-evident, that pancakes and waffles are good."

Just a Little Caution

Don't turn your waffle or pancake into a dessert! Nuts, nut butters, butter, margarine, and whipped cream are all high in fat. Also, many of these are bad for your arteries and heart. Use them sparingly, if at all, for greatest weight loss. Keep in mind that many pancake and waffle products contain little or no fiber. Be sure you read labels and buy only those that are whole grain.

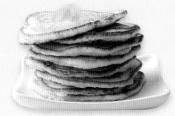

Getting Started

Let's face it—most of us don't have time in the morning to make waffles or pancakes from scratch. The good news is that it doesn't really take that long. There are many quick, easy-to-use products available—from frozen whole-grain waffles, which you can heat in the toaster, to easy-to-make pancake mixes using a variety of grains.

Good Foods from Your Store

Arrowhead Mills Organic Buckwheat Pancake & Waffle Mix	⅓ cup	7 g
Arrowhead Mills Organic Oat Bran Pancake & Waffle Mix	¼ cup	6 g

Toppings

Mott's Unsweetened Applesauce	½ cup	1 g
MaraNatha Almond Butter	2 Tbsp	4g

Homemade

If you decide to use a mix, or make from scratch, plan ahead and prepare a double batch. Freeze the leftovers—they reheat great. For a delicious power up, add chopped apple or blueberries to the batter before cooking.

DIANA'S FAVE

This is my favorite pancake/waffle topping because it's quick, easy, delicious, and loaded with fiber. I just soak 6–8 pitted dates in water until soft and put the dates and water in the blender. I add some fresh or thawed blueberries or blackberries and blend until not quite creamy. Then I pour this over a small bowl of the whole berries and mix all together. Sauce thickens within minutes as it sits.

Waffle/Pancake Fiber Wheel

Whole Grains

(Serving size = two 6" waffles or pancakes)
Multi-grain (10 g), Buckwheat (10 g),
Wheat (6 g), Spelt (8 g)

Toppings

(Serving size = 2 Tbsp)
Dried Fruit Puree (1 g),
Nut Butter (1 g),
Applesauce (1 cup) (4 g)

Fruit

(Serving size = 1 cup)
Blueberries (4 g),
Apple (chopped) (4 g),
Banana (sliced) (3 g),
Strawberries (sliced) (3 g)

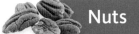

Nuts

(Serving size = 2 Tbsp)
Almonds (sliced) (1 g),
Walnuts (chopped) (1 g),
Pecans (chopped) (1 g),
Macadamias (1 g)

Dairy

(Serving size = ½ cup)
Yogurt (0 g),
Butter (1 Tbsp) (0 g),
Non-hydrogenated
margarine (1 Tbsp) (0 g)

FUN FACTS

Pasta is truly ancient. Archeologists have discovered 3000-year-old extruders for making pasta ribbons, later called "lagana" by the Romans, from which we take the word "lasagna." The Jewish Talmud tells us that cooking noodles was commonplace by 400 AD. Cortez, Balboa, Pizarro, and Ponce de León carried pasta to North and South America during the early 1500s. But the real genius, we think, is the unnamed hero who invented tomato sauce.

Getting Started

You have many choices. Lots of whole grains are used in pasta—everything from wheat, buckwheat, spelt, amaranth, quinoa, sprouted grains, rice—and many shapes are available, like elbow macaroni, fettuccine, spaghetti, angel hair, and shells. Whichever you choose, look for a fiber-rich product.

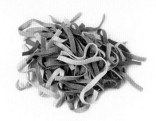

Good Foods from Your Store

DeBoles Organic Whole Wheat Spaghetti Style	2 oz	5 g
Bionaturae Organic 100% Whole Wheat Elbows	2 oz	6 g
Gia Russa 100% Whole Wheat Spaghetti and Penne	2 oz	5 g

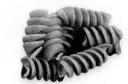

Pasta Sauce

Amy's Organic Family Marinara Pasta Sauce	½ cup	3 g
Ragu Robusto Roasted Garlic Pasta Sauce	½ cup	3 g
Newman's Own Marinara Sauce	½ cup	3 g

or

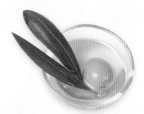

Homemade (serving for 2)

Add fresh or canned tomatoes (4 cups), tomato sauce (½ cup), onions, garlic (2 chopped cloves), other herbs, and extra-virgin olive oil (2 teaspoons). Add salt, lemon juice, fresh herbs, or Italian seasoning to taste.

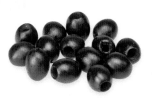

Just a Little Caution

Many store-bought sauces are high in calories, fat, and sodium. Consider making a batch of your own. It will keep for a few days in the fridge or you can freeze it.

DIANA'S FAVE

One of my favorite ways to power-up whole-wheat rotini is by adding soaked, sun-dried tomatoes that have been sautéed in extra-virgin olive oil with garlic, onions, and coarsely chopped kale. I mix the veggies with the cooked pasta, and add basil and salt to taste. Sometimes I throw in some cannellini or navy beans. Scrumptious!

Pasta Fiber Wheel

Whole Grains

(Serving size = 1 cup, cooked)
Whole Wheat (6 g), Multi-grain (4 g),
Ezekiel 4:9 Sprouted Grain (7 g), Buckwheat (3 g)

Sauces

(Serving size = ½ cup)
Marinara (3 g),
Fresh Tomatoes (chopped) (1 g),
Pesto (2 Tbsp) (2 g),
Olive Oil (2 Tbsp) (0 g)

Vegetables

(Serving size = ½ cup, cooked)
Broccoli (3 g),
Sweet Green Peppers (1 g),
Black Olives (2 g),
Mushrooms (2 g)

Fresh Herbs

(Serving size = 1 Tbsp, chopped)
Basil (0 g), Parsley (0 g), Garlic (0 g),
Chives (0 g)

Meat & Dairy

(Serving size = 3 oz)
Cheese (1 oz) (0 g), Chicken (0 g), Meatless
Burger Crumbles (4 g), Lean Ground Beef (0 g)

Beans

(Serving size = ½ cup, cooked)
Cannellini Beans (5 g),
Kidney Beans (6 g),
Black Beans (8 g),
Green Peas (5 g)

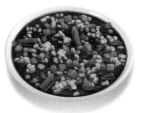

Getting Started

We don't have room to list all the possibilities, but here are a few delicious high-fiber combinations to try:

* Cold Gazpacho Soup—Vegetable juice, chopped raw carrots, sweet or spicy peppers, cucumber, and fresh cilantro
* Chili—Stewed tomatoes, beans, pasta, onion, peppers, and chili powder
* Lentil Stew—Broth, lentils, bulgur wheat, diced potatoes and carrots, and curry powder

The main difference between these dishes is the amount of broth, with soups having the most. Chili usually contains more beans, and since beans are the fiber giants, it is hard to go wrong with chili. But if you like soups or stews better, just include some beans and plenty of vegetables.

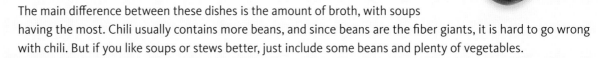

Good Foods from Your Store

Lakewood Super Veggie Vegetable Juice Blend	1 cup	4 g
Hunt's Stewed Tomatoes No Salt Added	1 cup	3 g
Imagine Organic No Chicken Broth	1 cup	0 g

Just a Little Caution

Canned soups usually are low in fiber and high in fat and salt—so be a good label detective. Or, better still, make your own healthy soup using the Fiber Wheel.

Soup/Chili/Stew Fiber Wheel

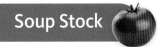

Soup Stock

(Serving size = 2 cups)
Vegetable Broth (0 g), Stewed Tomatoes (5 g),
Chicken Stock (0 g), Vegetable Juice (3 g)

Vegetables

(Serving size = 1 cup, raw)
Onion (chopped) (2 g),
Potatoes (cubed) (4 g),
Sweet Peppers (chopped) (2 g),
Carrots (fresh, sliced) (3 g)

Whole Grains

(Serving size = 1 cup, cooked)
Barley (6 g),
Bulgur Wheat (8 g),
Brown Rice (8 g),
Whole-Wheat Pasta Shells (5 g)

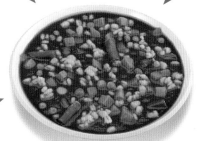

Herbs

(Serving size = 2 Tbsp, fresh, chopped)
Basil (0 g), Cilantro (0 g),
Parsley (0 g), Garlic (0 g)

Spices

(Serving size = 1 Tbsp)
Chili Powder (0 g),
Curry Powder (0 g), Cayenne (1 tsp) (0 g)

Meats

(Serving size = 3 oz)
Meatless Burger Crumbles (4 g), Chicken (0 g),
Lean Ground Beef (0 g), Baked Tofu (2 g)

Beans/Legumes

(Serving size = ½ cup, cooked)
Chili Beans (7 g), Lentils (8 g), Split Peas (8 g),
Green Beans (2 g)

Americans eat 350 slices of pizza every second; that's 100 acres of pizza a day. Evidently, we really like pizza. On October 11, 1987, Lorenzo Amato and Louis Piancone made a 44,457-pound pizza that covered 10,000 square feet. They cut it into 94,248 slices and served it to 30,000 happy people in Havana, Florida. In India, popular pizza toppings include pickled ginger, minced mutton, and tofu. The Russians prefer sardines, tuna, mackerel, salmon, and onions. No wonder we eat more pizza than they do.

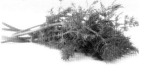

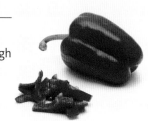

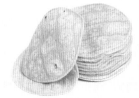

Getting Started

Nearly all pizzas at restaurants or in frozen food sections are made with processed grains, contain no fiber, and are usually high in fat and sodium. Here are some of the better grocery choices. No matter which crust you choose, be sure it has fiber.

Good Foods from Your Store

Whole Foods 365 Organic Whole Wheat Pizza Crust	¼ crust	3 g
Boboli 100% Whole Wheat Pizza Crust	⅕ shell	5 g
Trader Joe's Tabula Rasa Whole Grain Crust	⅛ crust	4 g

Pizza Sauces

Eden Organic Pizza Pasta Sauce—Italian Tradition	½ cup	5 g
Green Mill Classic Pizza Sauce	½ cup	2 g
Ragu Pizza Sauce—Homemade Style	½ cup	2 g

Homemade

To make an individual pizza, use a high-fiber tortilla or a whole-grain pita pocket as the crust. Toast for a few minutes in the oven, then add sauce and toppings, and bake until done.

Just a Little Caution

Cheese and meat products boost the fat and calories of pizza. Enjoy pizza flavor without sabotaging your weight-loss goals by leaving off the cheese and meat, or use them sparingly. The real flavor of pizza comes from the herbs, spices, and veggies.

One of my favorite create-your-own pizza options at a restaurant, or at home, is to substitute Bruschetta for pizza sauce. I get more fresh tomatoes, basil, and garlic with Bruschetta, plus the olive oil; then add spinach, broccoli flowers, and olives. Wonderful! When making a pizza at home, I love to replace pizza sauce with hummus, which gets a bit of a cheesy consistency when baked.

Pizza Fiber Wheel

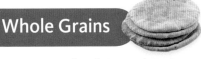

Whole Grains

Whole-Grain Pizza Crust (½ of 12" crust) (6 g),
La Tortilla Factory (1 Soft Wrap) (12 g),
Whole-Wheat Pita (6") (5 g)

Sauces

(Serving size = 1 cup)
Marinara (6 g),
Fresh Tomatoes
(chopped) (2 g),
Pesto (2 Tbsp) (2 g),
Olive Oil (2 Tbsp) (0 g)

Vegetables

(Serving size = ½ cup)
Black Olives (2 g),
Mushrooms (sliced) (0 g),
Bell Pepper (sliced) (1 g),
Onion (sliced) (1 g)

Herbs

**(Serving size = 2 Tbsp,
fresh chopped)**
Basil (0 g), Parsley (0 g),
Garlic (0 g), Oregano (0 g)

Beans

(Serving size = ½ cup)
Black Beans (cooked) (8 g),
Cannellini Beans (cooked) (5 g),
Hummus (8 g), Refried Beans (6 g)

Meat & Dairy

(Serving size = 3 oz)
Meatless Burger Crumbles (4 g),
Chicken (0 g), Cheese (1 oz) (0 g),
Soy Cheese (1 oz) (0 g)

FUN FACTS

The first recorded sandwich was made in Israel by Hillel the Elder in 20 BC when he put lamb and bitter herbs inside flat, unleavened bread during Passover. Seventeen-hundred years later, John Montagu, the fourth Earl of Sandwich, routinely ordered his valet to bring him meat tucked between two pieces of bread. Montagu was also a great supporter of Captain James Cook, who named the Sandwich Islands (now Hawaii) after him in 1778.

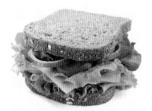

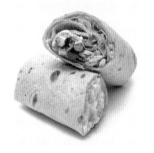

Just a Little Caution

Some sandwich spreads, such as mayonanaise, are high in fat and calories and have no fiber. Better choices are avocado, hummus, or nut butter.

Getting Started

If you are a sandwich lover and like densely packed fillers, use a meat slicer or vegetable mandolin to slice vegetables paper thin. Slice as many kinds of raw veggies as you want and stack between your bread with a dollop of your favorite sandwich spread and a sprinkle of oregano. Add a few leaves of fresh basil, and you will have a sandwich with more color and flavor than you ever imagined.

Good Foods from Your Store

La Tortilla Factory Soft Wraps	1 wrap	12 g
Orowheat Double Fiber Whole Grain Bread	1 slice	6 g
Rudi's Organic Bakery Multigrain Wrap	1 wrap	3 g
Toufayan 12 oz Whole Wheat Pita	1 pita	3 g

Spreads

Cedar's Hommus Tahini Original	2 Tbsp	1 g
Amy's Organic Refried Black Beans—Light in Sodium	½ cup	6 g

TERESA'S FAVE

I enjoy building a sandwich or wrap by starting with a foundation of dark leafy greens, then adding various vegetables or fruit. Thin layers are better than thick—they stack up better. A layer of onion, tomato, and shredded carrots is added to hummus, a veggie burger, or baked tofu. For interest, I may add a grain such as corn or pearled barley. A little sweetness can be dashed in by sprinkling dried cranberries, raisins, or currants. Fresh basil leaves, cilantro, oregano, or parsley can add a bit of zing to the lettuces or replace them altogether. I often dress the sandwich with avocado or homemade mayonnaise.

Pita/Sandwich/Wrap Fiber Wheel

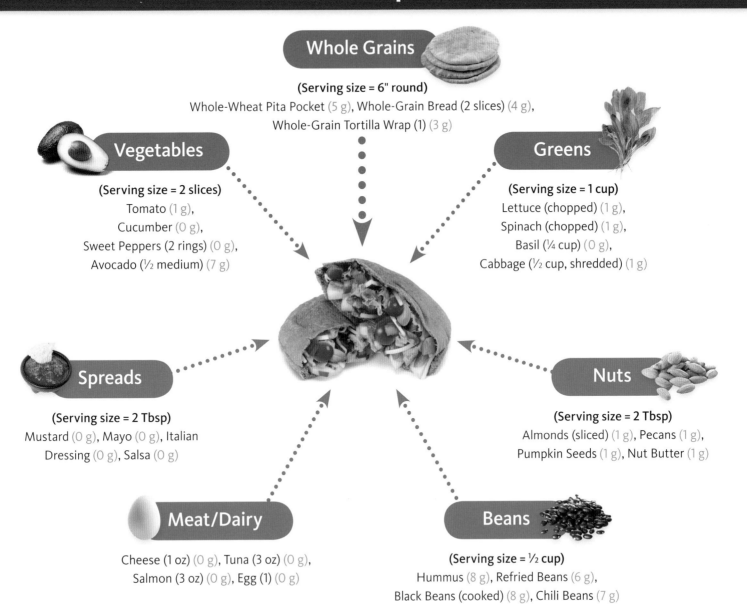

Whole Grains

(Serving size = 6" round)
Whole-Wheat Pita Pocket (5 g), Whole-Grain Bread (2 slices) (4 g),
Whole-Grain Tortilla Wrap (1) (3 g)

Vegetables

(Serving size = 2 slices)
Tomato (1 g),
Cucumber (0 g),
Sweet Peppers (2 rings) (0 g),
Avocado (½ medium) (7 g)

Greens

(Serving size = 1 cup)
Lettuce (chopped) (1 g),
Spinach (chopped) (1 g),
Basil (¼ cup) (0 g),
Cabbage (½ cup, shredded) (1 g)

Spreads

(Serving size = 2 Tbsp)
Mustard (0 g), Mayo (0 g), Italian
Dressing (0 g), Salsa (0 g)

Nuts

(Serving size = 2 Tbsp)
Almonds (sliced) (1 g), Pecans (1 g),
Pumpkin Seeds (1 g), Nut Butter (1 g)

Meat/Dairy

Cheese (1 oz) (0 g), Tuna (3 oz) (0 g),
Salmon (3 oz) (0 g), Egg (1) (0 g)

Beans

(Serving size = ½ cup)
Hummus (8 g), Refried Beans (6 g),
Black Beans (cooked) (8 g), Chili Beans (7 g)

FUN FACTS

Stephen J. Poplawski invented the blender in 1922. Seven minutes later he invented the smoothie. Today, Americans spend 2 billion dollars buying highly sweetened retail smoothies under the illusion that they're good for us.

TIP: When you order from a smoothie shop, tell them, "No turbinado." Turbinado is just a healthy-sounding name for SUGAR. Better yet, buy some fruit and make your own.

Getting Started

Buy fruit in season, when it is the sweetest and cheapest; ripe or over-ripe fruit can be frozen. When frozen fruit is blended to make a smoothie, the texture is almost like ice cream. You can also thicken smoothies and boost their fiber content by adding ground flaxseed, cashews, or a few tablespoons of mild-flavored beans. Smoothies are superior to fruit juices because they are powered-up with fiber.

Good Foods from Your Store

Blue Diamond Almond Breeze Original	1 cup	1 g
Silk Soymilk Original Unsweetened	1 cup	1 g
Dole Wild Blueberries (frozen)	1 cup	4 g
Dole Whole Strawberries (frozen)	1 cup	3 g

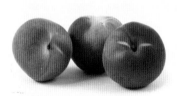

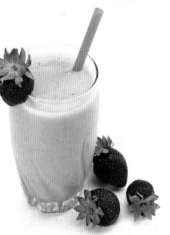

Just a Little Caution

It's fine to use dried fruits; they contain concentrated sugars and work well as a sweetener—dates, for example, are ideal. The downside—concentrated sugars = concentrated calories.

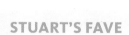

STUART'S FAVE

My favorite smoothie is great tasting, fiber-rich, and supercharged with antioxidants. Oh, and by the way, it's green. I simply blend fresh Swiss chard, frozen banana, and almond milk. It's a great way to start the day.

Smoothie Fiber Wheel

Liquid Base

(Serving size = 1 cup)

Almond Milk (0 g), Fruit Juice (unsweetened) (0 g),
Soy Milk (0 g), Low-Fat Milk (0 g)

Sweeteners

(Serving size = 1 Tbsp)
Dates (¼ cup) (3 g),
Agave Nectar (0 g),
Honey (0 g),
Fruit Juice Concentrate (0 g)

Fruit

(Serving size = 1 cup)
Berries (6 g),
Peaches (6 g),
Banana (3 g),
Pineapple (2 g)

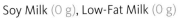

Nuts & Seeds

(Serving size = ¼ cup)
Cashews (1 g), Almonds (4 g),
Pecans (3 g), Flaxseed (2 Tbsp) (6 g)

Vegetables

(Serving size = 1 cup)
Swiss Chard (2 cups, chopped) (1 g), Carrots (shredded) (3 g),
Beets (shredded) (4 g), Celery (sliced) (2 g)

Flavorings

(Serving size = 1 tsp)
Vanilla Extract (0 g), Almond Extract (0 g),
Coconut Extract (0 g), Cinnamon (¼ tsp) (0 g)

Beans

(Serving size = ¼ cup, cooked)
Great Northern Beans (3 g), Navy Beans (5 g),
Cannellini Beans (3 g), Lima Beans (3 g)

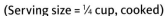

FUN FACTS

From its origins in Tibet, stir-frying spread into China, where it is done with peanut oil, ginger, and soy sauce, and India, where cooks prefer mustard oil, onions, and curry. Japanese chefs stir-fry with sesame oil, rice wine, and garlic. In Thailand, oil is avoided in favor of a watery stock, so the resulting food is light and bright. Serious enthusiasts worldwide recognize two distinctly different techniques: Chao, a low-heat sauté, and Bao, high-heat flash cooking.

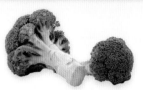
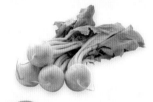
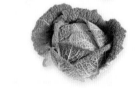
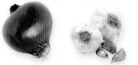
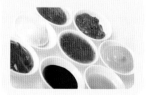

Just a Little Caution

It is easy to add lots of calories to stir-fry if you use too much oil or commercial sauces.

Getting Started

Stir-frys can be served on a bed of any whole grain, such as brown or wild rice, buckwheat noodles, barley, or quinoa. Quinoa is cooked much the same as rice.

Good Foods from Your Store

Ancient Harvest Quinoa	1 cup, cooked	5 g
Eden Foods Buckwheat Soba Noodles	1 cup, cooked	3 g
Whole Foods 365 Organic Shelled Edamame	½ cup	5 g

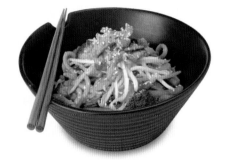

TERESA'S FAVE

When I stir-fry, I look for vegetables that hold their shape—sliced carrots, snow peas, sweet peppers, celery, broccoli, small squashes, green beans, even chopped greens like kale. Lots of onion and garlic are essential. Throwing in a few currants or cranberries can add a nice surprise. If you like heat, you can use ginger or cayenne. Cook quickly so that the veggies retain their bright colors. I usually steam them for a short burst, then spray with a small amount of oil to seal in color and crispness. Place the prepared vegetables over a bed of brown or wild rice and top with a tart dressing or peanut sauce. Eat with chopsticks for a change and a challenge! If you like finger foods, wrap it all in romaine lettuce.

Stir-Fry Fiber Wheel

Whole Grains
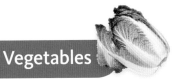

(Serving size = 1 cup, cooked)
Brown Rice (4 g), Buckwheat Noodles (3 g),
Quinoa (5 g), Wild Rice (3 g)

Fruit

(Serving size = ½ cup, fresh, chopped)
Pineapple (1 g), Mandarin Oranges (1 g),
Mango (2 g), Papaya (1 g)

Vegetables

(Serving size = 1 cup, sliced)
Carrots (3 g), Sweet Peppers (2 g),
Chinese Cabbage (1 g), Bamboo Shoots (3 g)

Flavorings
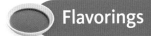

(Serving size = 2 Tbsp)
Low-Sodium Soy Sauce (0 g), Miso (0 g),
Bragg Liquid Aminos (0 g),
Toasted Sesame Oil (0 g)

Nuts & Seeds

(Serving size = ¼ cup)
Cashews (1 g), Sesame Seeds (4 g),
Pine Nuts (1 g), Peanut Butter (2 Tbsp) (2 g)

Meats

(Serving size = 3 oz)
Tempeh (6 g), Chicken (0 g),
Salmon (0 g), Lean Beef (0 g)

Beans/Peas

(Serving size = ½ cup, raw)
Snow Peas (1 g), Green Beans (2 g),
Edamame (3 g),
Garbanzo Beans (cooked) (6 g)

Herbs

(Serving size = ½ cup, fresh, chopped)
Cilantro (0 g), Basil (0 g),
Green Onion (2 g), Ginger Root (1 Tbsp) (0 g)

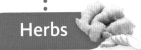

FUN FACTS

Every culture treasures its fruit salad. A salad of dried fruits and nuts is known as *khoshab* in the Middle East. *Rujak*, the spicy fruit salad of Indonesia, contains pineapple, mangoes, green apples, cucumber, black beans, chili paste, and lime. A Japanese fruit salad whose name we can't pronounce is made from lychees, pears, pineapple, peaches, and strawberries topped with instant coffee granules. Africans mix melons, apples, bananas, and oranges with cinnamon and vanilla. Yum!

Getting Started

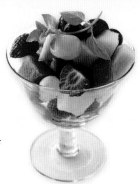

Chop or slice your favorite fruit(s), then top with granola, coconut, walnuts, macadamia nuts, pecans, pumpkin seeds, or flaxseeds. Mix in ½ cup of yogurt. For extra sweetness, add a dried fruit puree to any of the sauces listed on our Fiber Wheel. Soak dried fruits such as apricots, pears, mangoes, or dates in a small amount of hot water, then blend until smooth. Add water to get the consistency you desire. A small amount of puree goes a long way because of the concentrated sugar it contains.

Good Foods from Your Store

Silk Live Soy Yogurt Plain	½ cup	1 g
Nature's Path Organic Pumpkin Flax Plus Granola	¾ cup	5 g

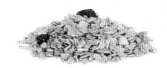 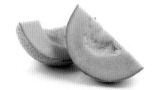 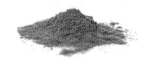

Just a Little Caution

Just because you are making a fruit salad doesn't mean you need to add whipped cream. It has no fiber and contains large amounts of fat and calories—makes it harder when you are trying to lose weight. Try one of the other sauces on our Fiber Wheel.

TERESA'S FAVE

To add a little extra sweetness, I put in a few raisins, dried cranberries, or currants. The colors and textures of sweet fruit, with crunchy nuts and chewy dried fruit, make it a treat. I buy fruit in season as much as possible in order to get the maximum flavor for the least price, sometimes splurging on items that are available only once a year. A container of blueberries is cheaper than going to the doctor.

Fruit Salad Fiber Wheel

Fresh Fruit

(Serving size = 1 cup)

Apples (chopped) (3 g), Berries (6 g),
Cantaloupe (chopped) (1 g), Kiwi (sliced) (5 g)

Sweeteners

(Serving size = 1 Tbsp)
Agave Nectar (0 g),
Fruit Juice Concentrate (0 g),
Fruit Jam (0 g),
Dried Fruit Puree (0 g)

Dried Fruit

(Serving size = 2 Tbsp)
Dates (chopped) (2 g),
Cranberries (1 g),
Coconut (shredded) (1 g),
Raisins (1 g)

Toppings

(Serving size = 2 Tbsp)
Almonds (slivered) (2 g),
Macadamia Nuts (1 g),
Pecans (1 g),
Granola (½ cup) (3 g)

Herbs & Spices
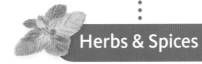

(Serving size = 1 Tbsp)
Fresh Mint Leaves (chopped) (0 g),
Candied Ginger (1 tsp, chopped) (0 g),
Cinnamon (sprinkle) (0 g), Nutmeg (sprinkle) (0 g)

Sauces

(Serving size = ½ cup)
Yogurt (0 g), Pureed Berries (3 g),
Fruit Juice (unsweetened) (0 g),
Smoothie (3 g)

Fiber Meal

See How the Fiber Adds Up

7 grams

6 grams

13 grams

TOTAL 26 grams

Fiber Meal

See How the Fiber Adds Up

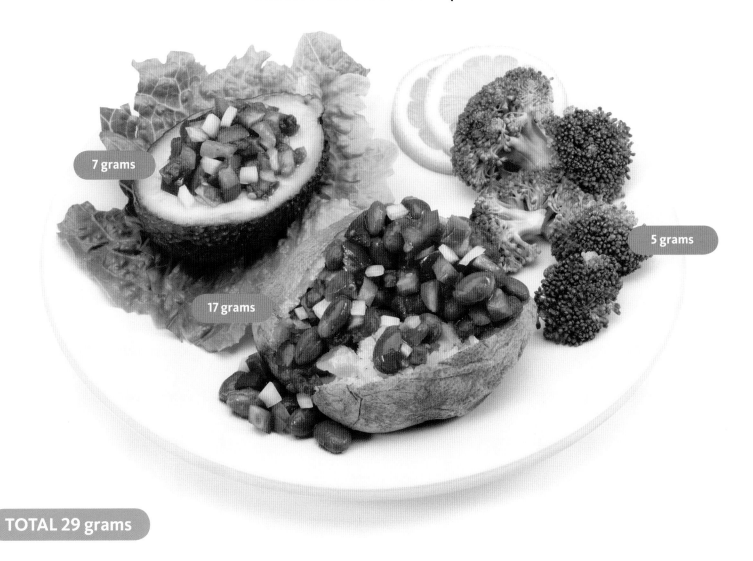

7 grams

17 grams

5 grams

TOTAL 29 grams

Taste Power Ups

CRUNCHY

almonds
sunflower seeds
apples
bell peppers
jicama
cucumber
celery
carrots
fennel

SWEET

raisins
dates
peaches
pears
pineapple or pineapple juice
bananas
grapes or grape juice
honey
agave nectar

ZINGY

salsa
chili peppers
cayenne pepper
curry/garam masala
paprika
mustard
ginger
lemon or lime juice
crushed red pepper

FLAVOR

roasted red peppers
lemon or lime
pico de gallo
pickle relish
garlic
basil
oregano
dill weed
extracts (vanilla, coconut, almond)

The Exchange

More This	Less That*
✔ Oranges	Orange Juice
✔ Brown Rice	White Rice
✔ High-Fiber Tortillas	White Flour Tortillas
✔ Whole-Grain Bread	White Bread
✔ Almonds	Candy
✔ Apples/Bananas	Cookies
✔ Sweet Potatoes	White Potatoes
✔ Berries	Brownies
✔ Oatmeal	Eggs
✔ Fruit Smoothies	Milk Shakes
✔ Beans or Hummus Dips	Sour Cream Dip
✔ Bran Muffins	Donuts
✔ Fruit Sorbets	Ice Creams
✔ Applesauce	Pudding
✔ Beans & Salsa on Baked Potatoes	Butter & Sour Cream on Baked Potatoes

* These have little or no fiber

STOP

CHALLENGE

CHOOSE

10 Weight-Loss Tips

1. Start every meal with fiber food and a glass of water.

2. Be aware of hunger. Quit eating when it's gone.

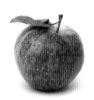

3. Seek vegetables. They love you unconditionally.

4. Put the silverware down between bites. Eat slower.

5. Leave food on your plate. It's okay.

6. If you're going to snack, pick a high-fiber food.

7. Fruits are your friends. Don't ignore them.

8. Start a Full Plate Diet club. Get skinny together.

9. Create high-fiber meals from restaurant menus.

10. Calories love Saturday. Be careful or they'll sneak up on you.

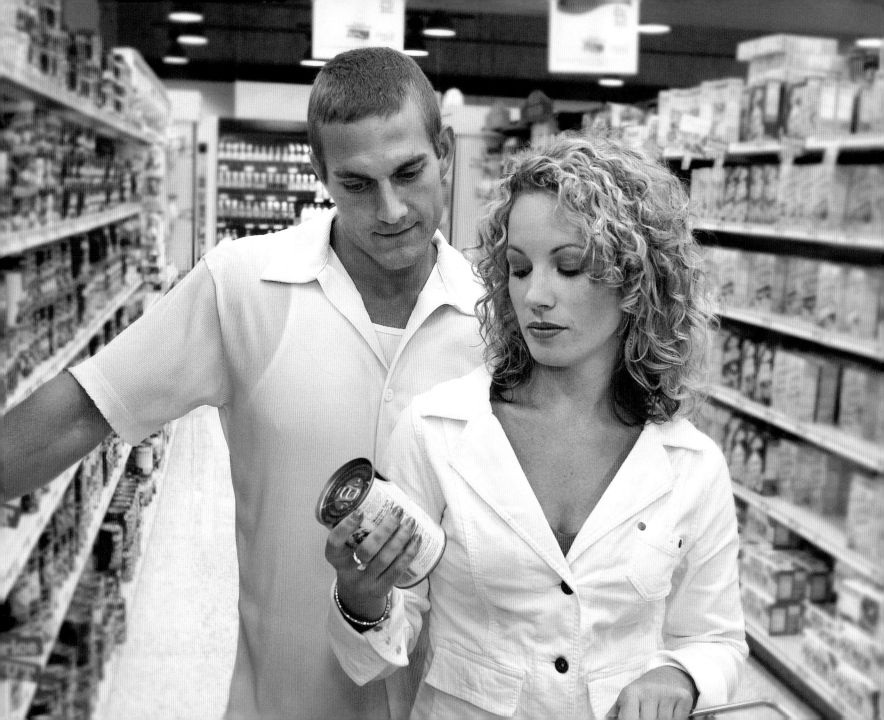

PART IV

Eating Smarter

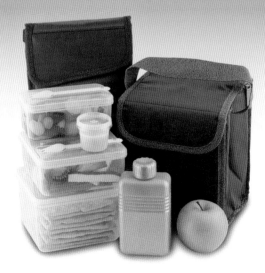

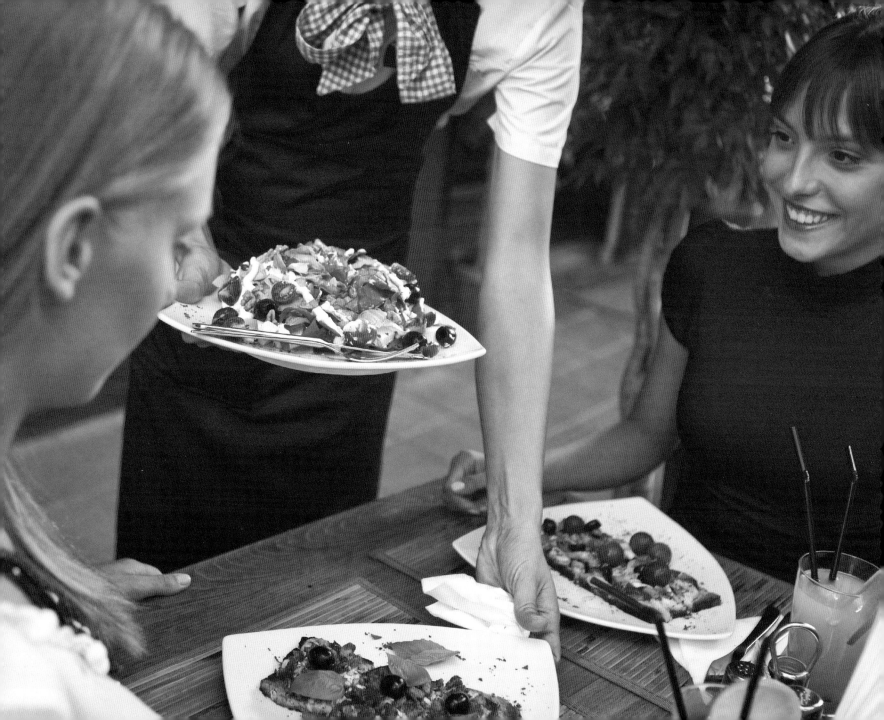

CHAPTER SEVEN

At the Office, Eating Out, & On the Road

Tell me what you eat, and I

will tell you what you are.

—Jean Anthelme Brillat-Savarin
  The Physiology of Taste

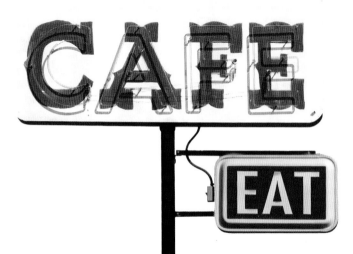

Lunch at the Office

Eat a high-fiber breakfast at home and you're happily on your way to 40 grams of fiber. Dinner will be a breeze. The trick is lunch. You can carry portable fiber foods, pack a brown bag, or make a quick and easy fiber meal in the kitchen at work.

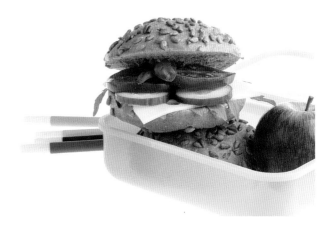

Office Kitchen

Many companies have a lunchroom with a refrigerator and microwave—not much, but enough to prepare a high-fiber meal or snack. You want a blender for making smoothies? Ask the boss if you can bring your own. And don't forget to drink plenty of water throughout the day. Most people get dehydrated at work, and thirst makes you eat too much.

Friends

In chapter 4 we mentioned the advantage of having friends join you on The Full Plate Diet—you can find new favorite foods together, give each other encouragement, and watch the pounds melt away. Talking makes you eat slower, and when you eat slower, you eat less.

Brown Bag

Bringing lunch from home gives you complete control of your fiber intake. If you eat plenty of fiber at lunch you'll be less hungry at dinner. The earlier you eat your calories, the more time you have to burn them before going to bed. Eat late and you'll add weight.

Temptations

The office is littered with tempting foods that have no fiber but are loaded with calories and chemicals that will make you unhappy. When a well-meaning friend brings a big box of donuts—Stop, Challenge, and Choose. Quick. Take a bite of an apple or a banana and feel that temptation fade.

Most Portable Fiber Foods

Raw veggies

Veggie or antipasto salad

Fresh fruit

Fruit salad

Bean salad

Whole-grain salad (such as tabouli)

Pita pocket with hummus & veggies

Whole-wheat veggie sandwiches

Bean or veggie wraps

Canned beans

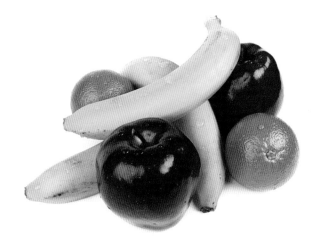

Birthday bashes and company parties are knee-deep in fattening foods. If you can't find any fiber and you want to be part of the party, just eat smaller portions and don't feel guilty. There will be other times for you to get your fiber. The secret is to minimize your portions. Remember, a tiny portion carries the same flavor as a big bite.

Take the edge off by eating a high-fiber food before the party, such as fresh fruit, veggies, or a big salad.

Quick & Easy Office Foods

High-fiber soups (lentil bean, vegetable, minestrone)

Baked sweet potato

Leftover brown rice with beans, other veggies

Smoothie (see chapter 6 for some ideas)

Whole-grain sandwich, pita, or wrap with fiber food

Yogurt with fresh fruit

Garden salad topped with canned beans and salsa

Eating Out

We don't expect you to use all of these suggestions, but do try to find a few that work for you. One big advantage of The Full Plate Diet is its infinite flexibility—that's what makes it sustainable. You might already be doing some of these things. If so, keep up the good work. Onward, to slimming down and looking great!

Restaurants

A restaurant menu isn't a problem, but a puzzle to be solved. And the prize for solving the puzzle is a slimmer, sexier you. There's always at least one high-fiber food on every menu, and some menus are simply loaded with them. When you're having a meal with a client or a group of friends, the temptation is to "join the crowd" when you order. This is a great time to—

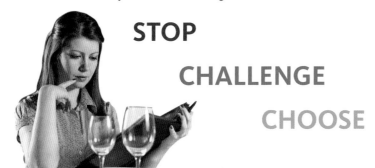

STOP

CHALLENGE

CHOOSE

Here are some tips

1. Select a restaurant with healthy menu options. Avoid buffets—you'll eat more when there's a greater variety of food available.

2. Plan ahead. Look up the restaurant online or call ahead to get menu information.

3. Beware of the bar. A cocktail while waiting to be seated can loosen your inhibitions and tempt you to order higher-calorie menu items.

4. Don't starve yourself before going out to eat. If you haven't eaten all day, you're much more likely to overeat. Drink a glass of water when you first sit down, and another before you order. This will reduce feelings of hunger, and you'll order less. Order a high-fiber starter, such as a salad, and eat it slowly before the rest of your meal arrives.

5. Divide your servings in half and share with a friend, or ask the waiter to bring a to-go box when your food is served, so you can halve your portion before you start eating.

6. Eat slowly. This will allow time for the fiber in your food to begin satisfying your brain's hunger center. You'll feel full faster and you'll eat less. Less food = more weight loss.

7. Be creative. Think of the menu as a list of ingredients available in the kitchen. If you see an item anywhere on the menu, it can be used to create a new menu option. Don't forget to look at the side dishes—many times there will be high-fiber foods you can use to power-up your entrée (for example: add steamed broccoli to your pizza or beans to your salad).

8. Ask for whole grains—whole-wheat pastas and bread, or brown rice. If your favorite restaurants don't carry them now, ask them to do so in the future.

9. Ask that your vegetables be steamed, baked, roasted, or grilled, not fried.

10. Going out to eat does not require you to have dessert—and in the long run you'll get more pleasure from not eating it and losing weight than from having a brief moment of taste-bud stimulation. If you feel the need for something sweet, order fresh fruit.

When you no longer feel hungry, stop eating. Leave it on your plate or ask for a take-out container.

On the Road

Business travel means eating at restaurants, so keep the tips above in mind. When flying, take food with you. Take another look at the Most Portable Fiber Foods in this chapter.

It's easy to put something good in a resealable plastic bag or plastic container and slip it into your briefcase. Not only will it taste better than airplane food, it's better for your figure. Airports are full of get-fat snacks: candy bars at the newsstands, aromatic cinnamon rolls, giant pretzels, ice cream. It's like a carnival. But things are slowly changing, and if you pay attention you may notice healthy fiber foods are available also. This is a wonderful time to Stop, Challenge, Choose—go for something you find that is healthy, or pull out your portable fiber food.

When driving, plan ahead by doing a restaurant search for places that promise options. In a pinch, let the "home cooking" restaurant fix you a vegetable plate instead of going to that burger place or fried chicken joint.

The key to eating on the road is a high-fiber breakfast. Most restaurants offer oatmeal, muesli, and other healthy grain dishes. Add some fresh fruit and you're off to a great start.

Onward!

One can not think well, love well, sleep well if one has not dined well.

—Virginia Woolf

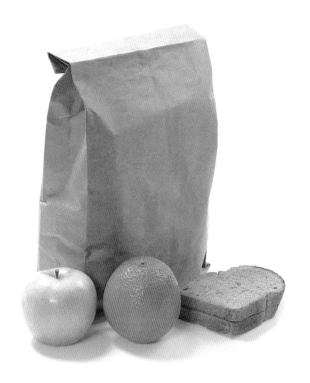

CHAPTER EIGHT

Become a
Nutrition Detective

If we're not willing to settle for
junk living, we certainly shouldn't
settle for junk food.

—Sally Edwards

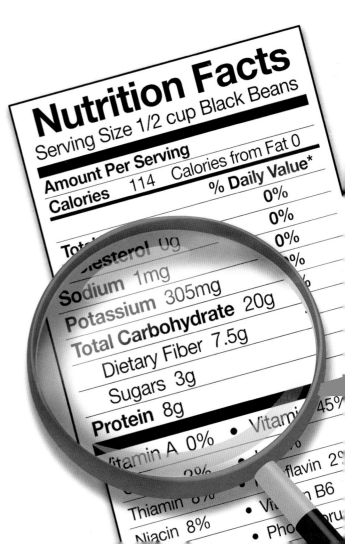

Nutrition Reports—3-Flag Ratings

Become a Detective

In chapter 3 we mentioned that Stage Three of The Full Plate Diet requires you to become a "label detective." To help get you get started, we made several trips to the grocery store to check random off-the-shelf product labels and obtained nutrition information from the web sites of fast-food and dine-in restaurants.

We came up with a 3-flag rating system—

Green means "go ahead." These foods can be eaten without sacrificing health or interfering with weight loss.

Yellow means "caution." These foods should be eaten in moderation or less frequently.

Red means "stop and think" before eating these foods. They will have a negative effect on your efforts to lose weight.

The following ratings aren't meant to be comprehensive. Our goal is merely to show you enough green, yellow, and red flags for you to recognize how we're arriving at these judgments—a starter list. These lists aren't meant to be a guide you carry with you to the grocery store. They're intended only to show you the things you should be looking for on nutrition labels and lists of ingredients.

Details of our rating system are at the end of this chapter.

At Your Grocery Store

Let's start with off-the-shelf products. There are a few generalities to keep in mind while grocery shopping. First, the more convenient a food has been made to prepare, the more likely it will be highly processed or otherwise loaded with unhealthy ingredients. The same is true for all snack foods. Read labels carefully. If you need help understanding the labels, visit **www.FullPlateDiet.org**.

Full Plate Diet Food Rating

Food Item	Rating	Reason
Bakery Goods		
Chips Ahoy! Chocolate Chip Cookies		Refined grain; Fat content; Added sugar
Nature Valley Granola Bars, Oats and Honey		Refined grain; Fat content; Added sugar
TLC Roasted Almond Crunch Bars		Refined grain; Fat content; Added sugar
Oreo Cookies		Sugar 1st ingredient; Refined grain; Fat content
Canned Beans / Bean Spreads		
Amy's Organic Refried Black Beans—Light in Sodium		
Eden Organic Great Northern Beans		
Westbrae Organic Pinto Beans		
Bush's Best Chili Beans Medium Sauce		Sodium 540 mg
Bush's Best Garbanzo Chick Peas		Sodium 470 mg
Bush's Best Pinto Beans		Sodium 450 mg
Cedar's Hommus Tahini Original		Fat Content
Van Camp's Pork and Beans in Tomato Sauce		Sodium 390 mg
Hormel Chili Turkey with Beans		Sodium 1250 mg
Canned Fruit		
Del Monte Tropical Fruit Salad (in 100% Juice)		
Dole Pineapple Chunks (in 100% Juice)		
Mott's Healthy Harvest No Sugar Added Applesauce		
Mott's Plus Fiber, Cranberry Raspberry		
Musselman's Natural Unsweetened Applesauce		
Del Monte No Sugar Added Sliced Pears		Artificial sweeteners
Del Monte Sliced Pears in Heavy Syrup		Added sugar
Dole Pineapple Chunks in Light Syrup		Added sugar
Musselman's Sweetened Applesauce		Added sugar
Del Monte Fruit Chillers, Polar Raspberry		Sugar 2nd ingredient
Ocean Spray Jellied Cranberry Sauce		Sugar 2nd ingredient

Full Plate Diet Food Rating (continued)

Food Item	Rating	Reason
Canned Vegetables		
Del Monte Fresh Cut Sliced Carrots		
Farmer's Market Organic Pumpkin		
Farmer's Market Organic Sweet Potato Puree		
S&W Julienne Carrots		
Del Monte Cut Green Beans—no salt added		
Del Monte Whole Kernel Corn—low sodium		
Del Monte Sliced Beets		
Hunt's Stewed Tomatoes		
Muir Glen Organic Italian Herb Pasta Sauce		
Amy's Organic Family Marinara Pasta Sauce		Fat content; Sodium 590 mg
Ragu Robusto Roasted Garlic Pasta Sauce		Fat content; Sodium 550 mg
Newman's Own Marinara Sauce		Sodium 510 mg; Added sugar
Eden Organic Pizza Pasta Sauce—Italian Tradition		Fat content
Green Mill Classic Pizza Sauce		Added sugar
Ragu Pizza Sauce—Homemade Style		Fat content
Del Monte French Style Green Beans		Sodium 390 mg
Del Monte Whole Leaf Spinach		Sodium 360 mg
Hunt's Diced Tomatoes		Added sugar
Bruce's Yams in Syrup		Added sugar
Del Monte Mixed Vegetables		Sodium 360 mg
Del Monte Peas and Carrots		Sodium 360 mg
S&W Petit Pois Peas		Sodium 360mg
Chips		
Guiltless Gourmet All Natural Tortilla Chips: Blue Corn, Yellow Corn, Chili Lime, Chile Verde, Unsalted Yellow Corn, Chipotle		
Fritos Original Corn Chips		Fat content
Mission Tortilla Triangles		Fat content; Refined grain

Full Plate Diet Food Rating (continued)

Food Item	Rating	Reason
Natural Tostitos, Original—Blue or Yellow Corn	🏴	Fat content
Rold Gold Classic Style Tiny Twists (pretzels)	🏴	Sodium 450 mg; Refined grain
Sun Chips Original, Multi Grain	🏴	Fat content
Doritos Spicy Nacho Chips	🏴	Contains MSG
Lay's Potato Chips, Classic	🏴	Fat content
Cold Cereals		
Cheerios	🏴	(Sugar 6g or less/serving)
Kashi GoLean	🏴	(Sugar 6g or less/serving)
Shredded Wheat Original	🏴	
Total, Whole Grain	🏴	(Sugar 6g or less/serving)
Wheaties	🏴	(Sugar 6g or less/serving)
Frosted Flakes	🏴	Refined grains; Added sugar
Special K	🏴	Refined grains
Fiber One Original	🏴	Artificial sweetener
Nature's Path Organic Pumpkin Flax Plus Granola	🏴	Fat content; Added sugar
Apple Jacks	🏴	Sugar 1st ingredient; Refined grain
Corn Pops	🏴	Sugar 2nd ingredient; Refined grain
Fruit Loops	🏴	Sugar 1st ingredient; Refined grain
Shredded Wheat Honey Nut	🏴	Sugar 2nd ingredient
Condiments & Pickles		
French's Mustard Classic Yellow	🏴	
Newman's Own Lighten Up Italian Dressing	🏴	
Pace Picante Sauce, Mild	🏴	
Vlasic Kosher Dill Spears	🏴	
Ortega Original Salsa	🏴	
Hunt's Catsup	🏴	
A1 Steak Sauce	🏴	
Hellman's Real Mayonnaise	🏴	Fat content

Full Plate Diet Food Rating (continued)

Food Item	Rating	Reason
Hidden Valley Ranch Original	🏴	Fat content; Contains MSG
Kikkoman Soy Sauce	🏴	Sodium 920 mg
Crackers		
Triscuits Original	🏳️	
Wasa Light Rye Crackers	🏳️	
Cheez-It Baked Snack Crackers	🏳️	Refined grain; Fat content
Kashi TLC Original 7 Grain Crackers	🏳️	Refined grain
Ritz Crackers	🏳️	Refined grain
Wheat Thins	🏳️	Refined grain; Fat content
Dairy Case		
Lisanatti Cheddar Style Almond Cheese	🏳️	
Lisanatti Mozzarella Style Almond Cheese	🏳️	
Blue Diamond Almond Breeze Original (almond milk)	🏳️	Fat content; Added sugar
Silk Live Soy Yogurt Plain	🏳️	Fat content; Added sugar
Horizon Organic Low Fat Milk	🏳️	Contains no fiber
Silk Soymilk—plain	🏳️	Fat content
Silk Soymilk—unsweetened	🏳️	Fat content
Kraft Shredded Colby & Monterey Jack Cheese	🏴	Fat content
Land O'Lakes Butter	🏴	Fat content
Fiber Bars		
Gnu Foods Flavor & Fiber Bars		
Orange Cranberry	🏳️	
Chocolate Brownie	🏳️	Added sugar
Fiber 35 Diet FitSmart Bars		
Lemon Poppy	🏳️	Added sugar
Cranberry Apple	🏳️	Added sugar
Fiber One Chewy Bars		
Oats & Chocolate	🏳️	Refined grain; Added sugar
Oats & Peanut Butter	🏳️	Refined grain; Added sugar

Full Plate Diet Food Rating (continued)

Food Item	Rating	Reason
Kellogg's FiberPlus Antioxidant Chewy Bars		
Chocolate Chip		Refined grain; Fat content; Added sugar
Dark Chocolate Almond		Refined grain; Fat content; Added sugar
Quaker Fiber & Omega 3 Bars		
Peanut Butter Chocolate		Refined grain; Added sugar
Dark Chocolate Chunk		Refined grain; Added sugar
South Beach Living Fiber Fit Granola Bars		
S'mores		Refined grain; Added sugar
Frozen Desserts		
Breyer's Natural Vanilla Ice Cream		Fat content
Breyer's Snickers Ice Cream		Fat content; Added sugar
Rainbow Popsicle		Added sugar
Luigi's Real Italian Ice, Cherry		Sugar 2nd ingredient
Mrs. Smith's Dutch Apple Crumb Pie		Trans fat
Frozen Entrees		
Boca Burger Original Vegan		
Morningstar Farms Burger Crumbles		
Lean Cuisine Vegetable Egg Roll		Refined grain; Sodium 620 mg
Morningstar Garden Vegetable Patty		Refined grain; Sodium 350 mg
DiGiorno Supreme Pizza		Refined grain; Sodium 1000 mg
Stouffer's Vegetable Lasagna		Refined grain; Sodium 980 mg
Frozen Fruits		
Dole Frozen Blueberries		
Dole Frozen Whole Strawberries		
Great Value WalMart Sliced Strawberries		Sugar 2nd ingredient
Frozen Vegetables		
Birds Eye Broccoli, Cauliflower & Carrots		
Green Giant Baby Sweet Peas		

Full Plate Diet Food Rating (continued)

Food Item	Rating	Reason
Whole Foods 365 Organic Shelled Edamame		
Green Giant Shoepeg White Corn & Butter Sauce		
Green Giant Broccoli, Carrots & Italian Seasoning		Fat content
Grain Products		
Ancient Harvest Quinoa		
Rudi's Organic Bakery Multigrain Wrap		
Toufayan 12 oz Whole Wheat Pita		
Whole Foods 365 Organic Whole Wheat Pizza Crust		
Trader Joe's Tabula Rasa Whole Grain Crust		
Arrowhead Mills Organic Buckwheat Pancake & Waffle Mix		
Arrowhead Mills Organic Oat Bran Pancake & Waffle Mix		
DeBoles Organic Whole Wheat Spaghetti Style		
Eden Foods Buckwheat Soba Noodles		
Bionaturae Organic 100% Whole Wheat Elbows		
Gia Russa 100% Whole Wheat Spaghetti and Penne		
La Tortilla Factory Soft Wraps		Added sugar
Orowheat Double Fiber Whole Grain Bread		Added sugar
Boboli 100% Whole Wheat Pizza Crust		Refined grain; Added sugar
Juices, Fruit		
Mott's 100% Apple Juice		
Welch's 100% Grape Juice		
Archer Farms (Target) Pink Peach Italian Soda		Added sugar
Diet Ocean Spray Cranberry Grape Drink		Artificial sweeteners (2)
Ocean Spray White Cranberry & Strawberry Drink		Sugar 2nd ingredient
Juices, Vegetable		
Archer Farms (Target) Tropical Carrot Juice		
Lakewood Super Veggie Vegetable Juice Blend		

Full Plate Diet Food Rating (continued)

Food Item	Rating	Reason
Archer Farms (Target) Vegetable Juice		Sodium 600 mg
Campbell's Tomato Juice		Sodium 680 mg
V8 100% Vegetable Juice		Sodium 480 mg
V8 100% Vegetable Juice—low sodium		Added sugar
Mott's Clamato Tomato Cocktail, original		Sodium 880 mg; Contains MSG
V8 Splash—Tropical Blend		Sugar 2nd ingredient; artificial sweetener
Margarines/Shortening		
Smart Balance Light		Fat content
Earth Balance Buttery Spreads		Fat content
Earth Balance Natural Shortening		Fat content
Nut Butters		
Earth Balance Natural Peanut Butter Crunchy		
Laura Scudder's Organic Peanut Butter Nutty		
Jif Natural Peanut Butter Creamy		
Smart Balance Peanut Butter Creamy		
Skippy Natural Peanut Butter		
MaraNatha Almond Butter		
Jif Reduced Fat Peanut Butter Creamy		Contains fully hydrogenated oil
Peter Pan Peanut Butter Creamy		Contains fully hydrogenated oil; Trans fat
Skippy Peanut Butter Creamy		Contains fully hydrogenated oil; Trans fat
Processed & Packaged Meat		
Ground beef patty		Fat content
Chicken, breast		Fat content
Salmon		Fat content
Turkey, ground patty		Fat content
Louis Rich Turkey Bacon		Fat content
Oscar-Mayer Bologna		Fat content
Tony Roma's World Famous Ribs		Sodium 910 mg; Trans fat
Mrs. Paul's Crunchy Fish Sticks		Trans fat

Full Plate Diet Food Rating

Food Item	Rating	Reason
Hillshire Farm Beef Smoked Sausage	🏴	Fat content; Trans fat
Oscar Mayer Lunchables Turkey & American Cracker Stackers	🏴	Sodium 870 mg; Trans fat
Snack Foods		
Crunchies Freeze Dried Mixed Fruit	🏳	
Crunchies Freeze Dried Strawberries	🏳	
Sun Maid Raisins	🏳	
Goldfish	🏳	Refined grain
Planter's Mixed Nuts	🏳	Fat content
Sun Chips Original	🏳	Refined grain; Fat content
Pringle's Original	🏴	Fat content; Refined grain
Soups		
Amy's Organic Lentil Vegetable	🏳	
Amy's Organic Chunky Tomato Bisque	🏳	Added sugar
Amy's Organic Low Fat Black Bean Vegetable	🏳	Sodium 430 mg
Campbell's Select Harvest Light Italian Style Vegetable	🏳	Sodium 480 mg
Imagine Organic No Chicken Broth	🏳	Sodium 450 g
Pacific Natural Foods Organic Creamy Butternut Squash	🏳	Sodium 550 mg
Progresso Chicken with Rice	🏳	Sodium 440 mg
Campbell's Chicken Noodle	🏴	Sodium 870 mg; Contains MSG
Campbell's Tomato	🏴	Sodium 790 mg; Added sugar
Progresso Lentil Soup	🏴	Sodium 870 mg
Progresso Light Italian Style Vegetable	🏴	Sodium 700 mg; Contains MSG

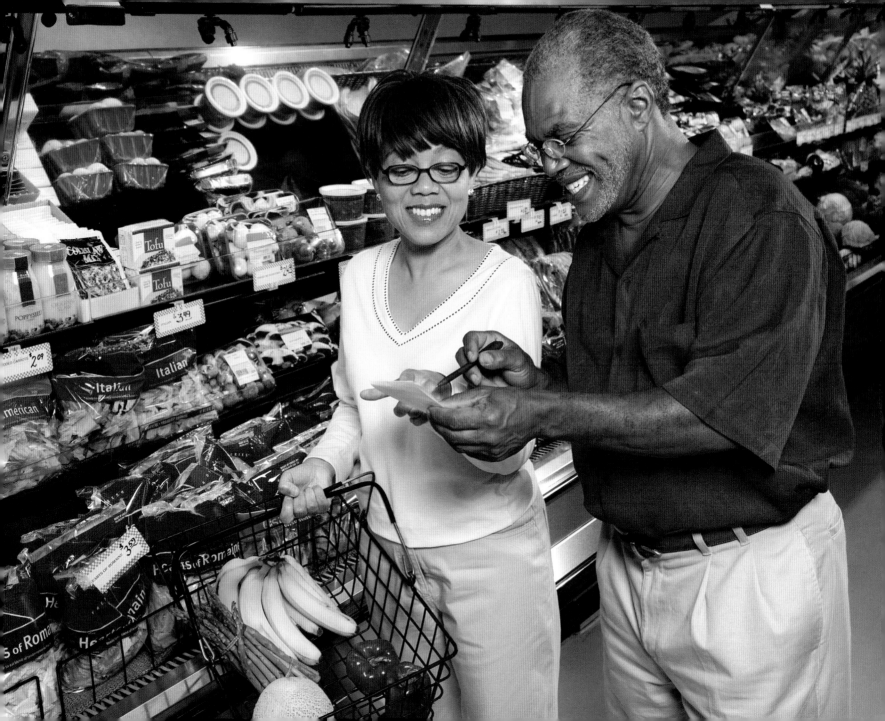

Eating Out

Most restaurants have few healthy food choices available. Restaurant foods are usually highly processed, contain large amounts of fat and sodium, and are high in calories. Because of this, we've given nearly all restaurant foods at best a "yellow." You're going to have to eat at restaurants. We know that. Compromise is an inescapable fact of life. The goal of the rating system is merely to give you a better sense of when your diet is on the bull's-eye and when it's a little off target.

Many national chain restaurants don't have nutritional information posted on their web sites. During our time online, we were unable to find complete nutritional info for a number of restaurants. If a restaurant chooses not to post nutritional information about its food, you've got to ask yourself why.

A good detective will plan ahead and visit the restaurant's web site, find the menu, and read the nutritional information.

Try to choose foods you can rate as "green." If you must choose "yellow" items, split portions with another person to minimize your exposure to unhealthy ingredients and/or concentrated calories. Sharing a dessert isn't as good as skipping dessert entirely, but it's twice as good as eating the whole dessert yourself.

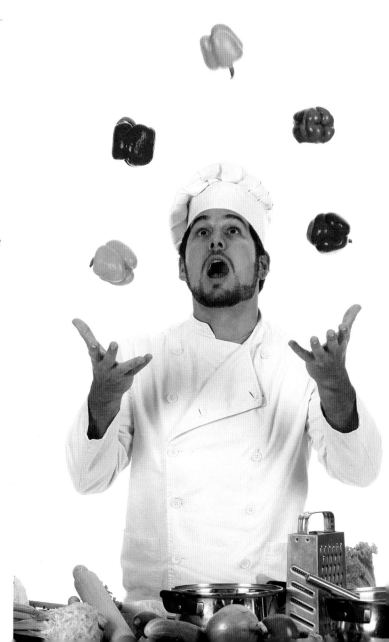

Fast-Food Rating

Restaurant	Menu Item	Rating	Reason	Tips to Improve Rating
Burger King	BK Fresh Apple Fries w/o caramel	🚩		
	Macaroni and Cheese	🚩	Refined grain pasta	
	Garden Salad w/Light Italian dressing	🚩	Sodium 550 mg	Cut dressing by ½ 🚩
	BK Veggie Burger w/o mayo	🚩	Refined grain bread; Sodium 1030 mg	
	Tendergrill Chicken Sandwich w/o mayo	🚩	Refined grain bread; Sodium 1130 mg	
Chili's	Guiltless Grilled Salmon	🚩	Sodium 420 mg; 46% total calories from fat	
	Grilled Salmon w/ garlic & herbs	🚩	46% total calories from fat	
	Buffalo Chicken Fajitas	🚩	Sodium 5260 mg; 65% total calories from fat	
KFC	3-Bean Salad	🚩		
	Corn on Cob, no butter	🚩		
	Cole Slaw	🚩	50% total calories from fat	
	Chicken Breast	🚩	Sodium 1050 mg	
	w/o skin or breading	🚩	Sodium 510 mg	
	Chicken and Biscuit Bowl	🚩	1 g trans fat; Sodium 2440 mg	
McDonald's	Premium Southwest Salad, no dressing	🚩		
	w/Newman's Southwest dressing	🚩	Sodium 490	Cut dressing by ½ 🚩
	w/Newman's Ceasar or Ranch dressing	🚩	Sodium 650 to 680 mg, depending on dressing	
	w/any other dressing	🚩	Sodium 880 to 890 mg	Cut dressing by ½ 🚩

* All burgers from the fast food restaurants are rated RED because of refined grain bread, trans fat, high fat calories, and high sodium

Restaurant	Menu Item	Rating	Reason	Tips to Improve Rating
	w/crispy chicken & any dressing	🏴	Sodium 1260 to 1660 mg, depending on dressing	
	Filet-O-Fish Sandwich	🏳	Sodium 640 mg; refined grain bun	
	Medium Fries	🏳	45% total calories from fat	
	Egg McMuffin	🏴	Sodium 820 mg	Get plain muffin 🏳
	Quarter Pounder w/o cheese*	🏴	1 g trans fat	
Papa John's	The Works, 14" Original Crust, 1 slice	🏳	Refined grain crust; Sodium 890 mg	
	Garden Fresh, 14" Whole Wheat Crust	🏳	Sodium 660 mg	No olives, cheese 🏳
P.F. Chang's	Sweet and Sour Chicken	🏳	39% total calories from fat	
	Stir Fried Eggplant	🏳	Sodium 438 mg	
	Beef with Broccoli	🏴	Sodium 2159 mg	
Red Lobster	½ portion of any fresh fish, except Arctic Char or Cobia; broiled or grilled, with broccoli, and no Chef's Spices or Sauces	🏳		
	Full portion of Sole, Tilapia, or Cod; broiled or grilled, with broccoli, and no Chef's Spices or Sauces	🏳		
	Blackened Catfish	🏳	43% total calories from fat	
	Shrimp Linguine Alfredo	🏴	Sodium 3160 mg	

Restaurant	Menu Item	Rating	Reason	Tips to Improve Rating
Romano's Macaroni Grill	Spaghetti & Meat Balls	🚩	Sodium 4900 mg	
	Chicken Portobello	🚩	Sodium 3140 mg	
Subway	Veggie Delight Salad	🏳		
	w/ Ranch Dressing	🏳	Sodium 635 mg	Cut dressing by ½ 🚩
	w/Low Fat Italian	🚩	Sodium 795 mg	Cut dressing by ½ 🏳
	6" Veggie Delight Sandwich	🏳	Refined grain bread; Sodium 500 mg	
	6" Turkey Breast	🚩	Refined grain bread; Sodium 1200 mg	
	Veggie Delight Wrap	🚩	Refined grain wrap; Sodium 750 mg	
Taco Bell	Chalupa Supreme—Steak	🏳	48% total calories from fat; Sodium 530 mg	
	Beef Burrito Supreme	🚩	Refined grain tortilla; 1 g trans fat; Sodium 1350 mg	
	Fresco Bean Burrito**	🚩	Refined grain tortilla; 0.5 g trans fat; Sodium 1200 mg	
	Grilled Stuft Burrito—Chicken	🚩	Refined grain tortilla; 0.5 g trans fat; Sodium 2160 mg	
	Fiesta Taco Salad w/o shell	🚩	1.5 g trans fat; Sodium 1520 mg	
Wendy's	Baked Potato	🏳		
	w/broccoli & buttery spread	🏳		
	w/broccoli & cheese	🏳	Sodium 450mg	
	w/bacon pieces	🏳	Sodium 530 mg	
	w/bacon pieces & cheese	🚩	Sodium 950 mg	
	¼ lb Single Burger	🚩	Refined grain bread; 1 g trans fat; 42% total calories from fat; Sodium 870 mg	
	Southwest Taco Salad	🚩	55% total calories from fat; Sodium 1570 mg; 1 g trans fat	Remove strips; fat-free Ranch 🏳

** Taco Bell refried beans contain trans fat, except in New York City

Suggestions for Avoiding Trans Fat

Remember: Hydrogenated and "partially hydrogenated" oil and shortening are trans fat.

1. **Avoid deep-fried foods**
* partially hydrogenated oil is used for deep frying

2. **Salad dressings**
* ask if the salad dressing is made with partially hydrogenated oil
* use lemon juice and/or olive oil
* bring your own

3. **Watch out for those dinner rolls!**
* they're usually made with partially hydrogenated oil. And if you don't eat the rolls, you won't need the butter (high in saturated fat) or the margarine (usually contains partially hydrogenated oil)

4. **Go easy on the crackers**
* they're almost always made with partially hydrogenated oils

5. **Avoid cakes, pies, donuts, and other pastries**
* they're loaded with shortening and/or partially hydrogenated margarines and oils. (You didn't really think we were going to give donuts a green flag, did you?)

Food Sources

Think of these as general guidelines when evaluating food:

1. Grown organically and fresh from your own garden. BEST! Happy, Happy, Happy.

2. Organically grown, farmer's market or store-purchased. GREAT! Happily dancing.

3. Grown non-organically in your garden. Still GREAT!

4. Farmer's market or store-fresh veggies & fruits, with selected whole-grain breads and cereals, beans, and nuts. VERY GOOD.

5. Canned and frozen fruits, veggies, and beans without added fat, salt, or sugar. GOOD. Much better than the average American diet.

6. Carefully selected restaurant foods. GOOD. Sort of.

7. Canned and frozen fruits, veggies, and beans with fat, salt, or sugar added. BAD.

8. Junk restaurant food. VERY BAD.

9. Junk snack food & drinks. EXTREMELY BAD. You may fall over dead before you eat that last bite. Just looking at the wrapper has been known to cause blindness. (You know we're kidding, right? Still, snack foods are very unhappy.)

Beyond Fiber

Increase your dietary fiber and you'll experience numerous health benefits, one of which is sustainable weight loss. Seek out foods that are high in fiber. The nutritional quality of a food, however, is more than just how much fiber it contains. This is especially true when it comes to commercial food products. A whole-plant food is the gold standard. Whole-plant foods are wholly derived from plants, and as close as possible to the way they came off the vine or tree, or out of the ground. Shop in the produce section and you'll lose weight.

Packaged foods are a different story. Some packaged products offer high nutrition, have very little processing, and use only a few ingredients. These are the ones you should eat. For grain products, you should see the words "whole grain." Other packaged products have numerous ingredients or are processed with additives that make them less healthy. Try to avoid products containing white or "enriched" flour, fats, sugars, or artificial sweeteners.

The worst foods are highly processed and include ingredients that are extremely unhealthy. These should be avoided completely. Watch out for trans fat and monosodium glutamate (MSG), and foods that have high-fructose corn syrup or sugar as the first or second ingredient on the list. (By federal law, an ingredient list must show the highest volumes at the top of the list. The closer an ingredient appears to the top of the list, the more of it is in the food.)

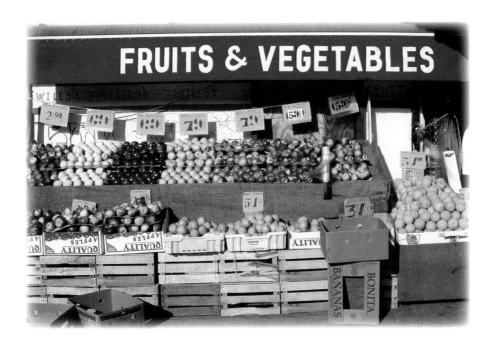

Details of Our Rating System

Green

* All whole-plant foods. Those that contain high amounts of fat, such as coconut, avocado, nuts, seeds, and nut butter, should be eaten in moderation if you want to lose weight faster
* Commercial or restaurant items that contain:
  – 100% whole grains (no white or enriched flour)
  – Sodium less than 350 mg per serving
  – Calories from fat less than 25% of the total
  – No trans fat, MSG, artificial sweeteners (aspartame, sucralose, saccharin, or acesulfame)
  – No added sugars (high-fructose corn syrup, dextrose, evaporated cane juice, etc.)

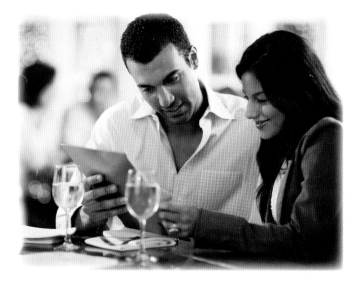

Yellow

* Red meat, pork, poultry, fish, and most dairy products (milk, cheese, yogurt, ice cream, etc.), and eggs
* Commercial or restaurant items that contain:
  – Processed grains
  – Sodium between 350 mg and 750 mg per serving
  – Calories from fat between 25% and 60% of the total
  – Artificial sweeteners
  – Added sugars

Red

* Commercial or restaurant items that contain:
  – MSG
  – Added trans fat
  – Fat calories more than 60% of the total
  – Sodium more than 750 mg per serving
  – Added sugars first or second on the ingredient list

If you're aware of what you eat, and what's in what you eat, you'll live a longer, happier, healthier life. And you'll slim down and look great, too. That's our **wish** for you.

CHAPTER NINE

A Little Medical Talk

Let food be your medicine and medicine be your food.

—Hippocrates

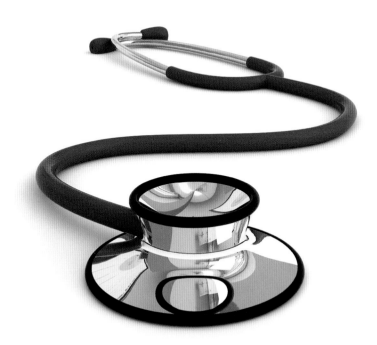

A Little Medical & Nutrition Talk

You probably bought this book because you want to look better. You're definitely going to get that from it. The mirror is going to love the new you.

Hopefully, what you've read has caused you to become a little more interested in living a healthy lifestyle. Vigor, vitality, stamina, and optimism flow from a healthy body.

Prior to publishing this book, we gave a few hundred advance copies to readers and asked them to submit any questions they might have.

Here's what we got.

Audience Qs

1. **So, what's the big fuss about trans fat? I get confused sometimes. There's polyunsaturated fat and trans fat. What's the difference?**

A: Trans fats are detrimental to health because they increase your "bad" cholesterol and lower "good" cholesterol levels in your body. Trans fats promote blockage of your arteries, thus increasing your risk for heart attack, stroke, and other vascular diseases. Trans fat is called "partially hydrogenated oil" or "shortening" in the ingredient list. Polyunsaturated fat, on the other hand, is healthy and helps prevent blood vessel disease. Vegetable oils are an excellent source of these beneficial fats, provided they've not been hydrogenated or partially hydrogenated.

2. **What about artificial sweeteners?**

A: There's conflicting research regarding the effects of artificial sweeteners. As of this writing, it is our opinion that natural sweeteners are a better choice, and the use of artificial sweeteners should be limited until conclusive research is available.

Follow up Q: What substitutes do you recommend?

A: Honey is a readily available natural sweetener. Agave nectar, made from the agave cactus, is also an excellent substitute. These sweeteners are much better for you than table sugar, but they should still be used in moderation.

3. Why should I care about sodium? Is it the same as salt?

A: Most Americans consume at least twice the daily maximum recommended amount of sodium, which is 10 to 20 times the amount necessary to sustain life. Most of this sodium is from salt which is added to processed foods. Sodium raises blood pressure, a major risk factor for heart attack, stroke, kidney failure, and blindness.

4. Do I need to continue taking supplements like B-6, omegas, and minerals if I'm eating lots of fiber?

A: One of the beautiful things about fiber-rich foods is that they're also packed with vitamins, essential fatty acids, minerals, antioxidants, and phytochemicals. Most supplements are unnecessary when you eat The Full Plate Diet, unless you're taking special supplements under the guidance of your physician.

5. I've noticed several new products that advertise high fiber. Are these for real, or are they just processed food in disguise?

A: The best way to increase dietary fiber is to eat whole-plant foods as unprocessed as possible. Some manufacturers are adding fiber to their processed foods but it's not yet clear if this added fiber is as beneficial as naturally occurring fiber. If a product is essentially unhealthy, it will still be unhealthy if you add fiber. Fiber isn't magic, it's merely a marker for foods that contain vitamins, essential fatty acids, minerals, antioxidants, and hundreds of important phytochemicals that can be obtained no other way.

6. How can I use The Full Plate Diet to help control my diabetes?

A: Fiber is a great way to help control blood sugar, and losing weight is also critical. This diet will help you do both. If you want to stop, and possibly reverse, type 2 diabetes, you need to count carbs, limit high glycemic foods, get regular physical activity, check your blood sugar routinely, eat meals at a consistent time every day, manage stress, and get adequate rest. If you want help in any or all of these areas, call 877-775-2610, or go to **www.FullPlateDiet.org**.

7. There's been a lot of advertising for green tea and acai. I assume they have no fiber, but are they good? Or is it all hype?

A: You're right, teas and juices don't contain fiber but they do often contain other beneficial nutrients. Green tea and acai are sources of healthy antioxidants. But if you eat a variety of fiber-rich foods such as are in The Full Plate Diet, you'll get these antioxidants, plus the benefits of fiber, too.

8. What does sugar do to us?

A: Most carbohydrates are eventually broken down and converted into "blood sugar," which is the body's basic fuel. For blood sugar to become energy, the pancreas must secrete insulin to allow the sugar to enter our cells. Refined, "simple" carbohydrates like table sugar are easily digested and rapidly absorbed, making the pancreas work very hard to move the blood sugar into the cells. Added sugars in foods overwork our organs. Unprocessed foods containing natural sugars almost always contain fiber. This slows the absorption of the sugar, causing much less stress to the body.

Follow up Q: Is corn syrup the same as sugar?

A: Corn syrup (HFCS) is not technically the same compound as table sugar (dextrose) but it's almost as bad for you. Corn syrup is especially prevalent in juices, soft drinks, and other processed or snack foods. Avoid it if you can.

9. The Full Plate Diet allows me to eat meat and dairy products if I choose, but health-wise, does it make a difference?

A: Meat and dairy products are high in harmful saturated fat, low in antioxidants, and contain zero phytochemicals and fiber. Additionally, meat and dairy products are high in calories per volume of food and very likely high in toxins due to pesticides, antibiotic residues, and growth hormones. These nasty chemicals are the opposite of antioxidants, contributing to heart attack, stroke, high blood pressure, high cholesterol, cancer formation, osteoporosis, antibiotic sensitivities, and bacterial antibiotic resistance. The lower your consumption of meat and dairy products, the better your health will be.

Follow up Q: How about fish, isn't it supposed to be high in omegas?

A: Fatty fish like salmon contain omega-3 essential fatty acids. The major problem with fish is that the pollution of our oceans has contaminated most fish with heavy metals, pesticides, chemical dyes, and other toxins. These problems are probably manageable if your fish consumption is occasional, but a steady diet of fish is becoming questionable. Fish get their omega-3 fatty acids from marine algae—a green "vegetable," so to speak. Likewise, you can get omega-3 fatty acids by eating green leafy vegetables, nuts, and seeds. Ground flaxseed and walnuts are good sources of omegas.

10. What about fiber supplements—will they help me lose weight?

A: Research shows that increasing your fiber intake helps you lose weight, even if the fiber comes from a supplement. While it is more desirable to get your fiber from food, this is not always easy to do, such as when traveling or at the office. In those instances you can consider using a supplement such as Metamucil, Metamucil Clear and Natural (previously known as Fibersure), or Citrucel. If you use these products, do not exceed the serving size recommendations.

11. I know this is a silly question, but is chocolate good or bad for you? I've heard both.

A: Ah, if only it were that simple! Imagine how many books we'd have sold if this had been called *The Chocolate Diet*. Cacao (cocoa) beans are high in beneficial antioxidants. However, they're also more than 50% fat. And we never eat these cacao beans raw. We add sugar, fat, and milk. Like other things, a little dark chocolate from time to time is okay, but eating it every day is a bad idea.

12. Is it okay to drink beer and wine?

A: There's research to indicate that drinking one serving per day of beer or wine may be beneficial in reducing heart attacks. Other studies show a definite link between alcohol consumption in any amount and an increase in certain cancers in women. Also, as we mentioned earlier, alcohol lowers inhibitions, which often leads to more eating.

13. Sometimes when I eat sweets or drink alcohol or coffee, I need to take an antacid. What's happening?

A: Sweets, alcohol, and coffee contain irritating acids and they also stimulate the stomach to over-produce its own acid. This causes stomach acids to get up into the esophagus where they don't belong. This problem is accelerated if you overeat or you're overweight. Lying down too soon after you eat also contributes to the problem. Stomach acid in the esophagus is called heartburn or sour stomach. Thus, the antacids.

Follow-up Q: So how do I stop it?

A: Your body is telling you to quit eating or drinking the offending foods, especially within 4 hours of lying down to sleep. The Full Plate Diet has been shown to reduce and eliminate heartburn and sour stomach. Try it.

For more information, please visit **www.FullPlateDiet.org**.

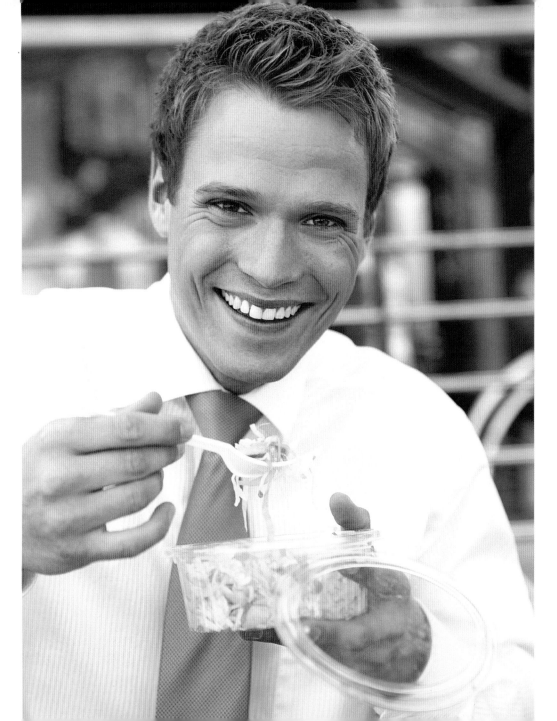

No one can
cheat you out of
ultimate success
but yourself.

—Ralph Waldo Emerson

CHAPTER TEN

Onward!

The most difficult thing is the decision to act, the rest is merely tenacity. The fears are paper tigers. You can do anything you decide to do.

—Amelia Earhart

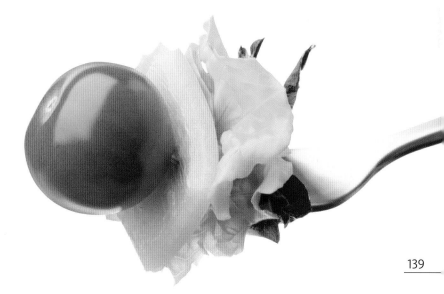

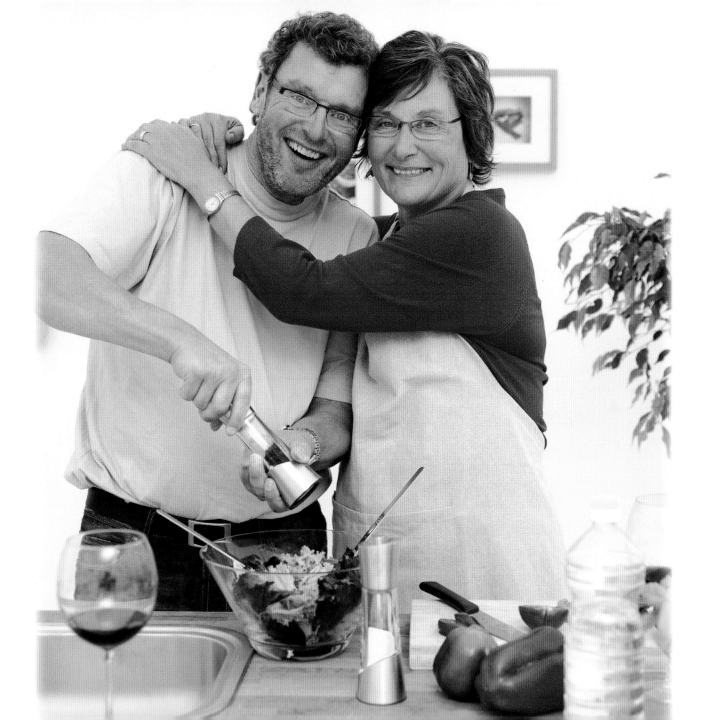

Dear Reader,

You're it. You're the one. It's you.

No one else has the authority to decide how you'll think, look, and feel.

What have you decided?

We want—very much—for you to love being alive. Health, energy, and a positive self-image are wealth beyond words.

We wrote this book to give those things to you.

You thought we did it for the money? What money? The authors' royalties from this book will go to a non-profit organization. We wanted it that way.

We didn't write this book to make money. We wrote it to make a difference in *your* life.

You. You're the one.

We've shared these financial details only to strengthen your confidence in our motives and hopefully, lift your spirit. We desperately want you to know how special you are.

We have confidence in you.

You can do this!

ONE LAST TIME: Eat 40+ grams of fiber each day, begin every meal and snack with fiber foods, drink more water, and don't eat when you're not hungry—and your life will change. It's as simple as that.

Cutting out just 350 calories per day translates to 35 pounds of weight loss in a year. And if you're eating high-fiber foods, you'll never miss those calories. Take the stairs instead of the escalator and your results will happen even faster.

Did you know The Full Plate Diet is thousands of years old? The earliest record of it is found in the first chapter of the book of Daniel. Medical historians consider it to be the world's first clinical trial of a diet:

> When Daniel asked that he and Shadrach, Meshach, and Abednego be exempted from eating the food provided by the king of Babylon, the guard replied, "I am afraid of my lord the king, who has assigned your food and drink. Why should he see you looking worse than the other young men your age? The king would then have my head because of you." Daniel then said to the guard, "Please test your servants for ten days: Give us nothing

but vegetables to eat and water to drink. Then compare our appearance with that of the young men who eat the royal food, and treat your servants in accordance with what you see." So the guard agreed to this and tested them for ten days. At the end of the ten days they looked healthier and better nourished than any of the young men who ate the royal food. So the guard took away the food and the wine they were to drink and gave them vegetables instead.

Just as Daniel had to gain the cooperation of the guard sent by the king of Babylon, you'll have to deal with well-meaning friends, family, and co-workers. Will you know what to say when someone who loves you announces she made your favorite brownies? And how will you respond to the friend who's convinced you're not getting enough protein? Sadly, the biggest problem often occurs after the pounds begin to noticeably drop off. That's when jealousy and fear can show up in the attitudes of the people nearest you. These loved ones are going to need reassurance that the new you is going to continue loving the old them.

Now is the time to begin thinking about these things. Remember: If you fail to plan, you plan to fail. Develop a plan for dealing with every potential setback. Win the support of the people around you. You might even inspire a few of them to follow in your footsteps.

Never forget you can do this. The Full Plate Diet is easy, fun, healthy, and it works. You're going to lose weight, feel younger, look better, and regain lost vitality.

We foresee a healthy, happy you.

Send us an email to let us know of your success. You can do this.

Stuart A. Seale, M.D.

Teresa Sherard, M.D.

Diana Fleming, Ph.D, LDN

About the Authors

Stuart A. Seale, M.D.

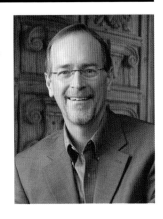

Stuart A. Seale, M.D., board-certified family physician and coauthor of *The 30-Day Diabetes Miracle* (Penguin, New York 2008) has helped thousands of patients over the past quarter century. While managing a solo family practice in Springfield, Missouri, for 21 years, he treated an increasing number of patients who suffered from lifestyle-related diseases, including obesity. This experience encouraged him to learn more about treating the cause of these conditions, not just how to control the symptoms.

He now serves as the medical director for Ardmore Institute of Health and is the medical director, physician, and educator for Lifestyle Center of America's diabetes and weight management programs in Sedona, Arizona.

Dr. Seale graduated from Loma Linda University School of Medicine in 1979 and completed a family practice residency at the University of Missouri in 1983. He has received the 3-year AMA Physician Recognition Award 8 times, most recently in 2007.

Diana Fleming, Ph.D., L.D.N.

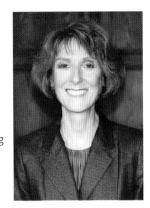

Diana Fleming, Ph.D., was cofounder and comanager of Country Life Vegetarian Restaurants in New York City and London and a cooking consultant for Harvard University and Wellesley College. She earned her Ph.D. in nutrition at Tufts University in Boston. All four of her thesis papers were published in the *American Journal of Clinical Nutiriton*.

Diana coauthored *The 30-Day Diabetes Miracle Cookbook* (Penguin, New York 2008), where her knowledge and expertise were valuable in developing tasty high-fiber, plant-based recipes that help readers achieve significant diabetes relief and weight loss.

She joined the staff at the Lifestyle Center of America in 2002, serving as Director of Nutritional Services since 2003. Too often nutrition professionals don't know how to take the theory of nutrition from research to the plate. Not so with Diana. She has a passion for nutrition which translates into her personal love for cooking, baking, and eating.

Teresa Sherard, M.D.

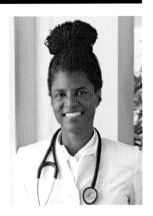

Teresa Sherard, M.D., earned her medical degree from Loma Linda University School of Medicine in 1999. She completed her internship and residency at Loma Linda University Hospital in 2002. Two years later, she completed a fellowship in lifestyle medicine at the Lifestyle Center of America.

As a staff physician at the Lifestyle Center of America, Dr. Sherard educates patients to recapture their health and to successfully achieve weight loss. This is accomplished when nutrition, exercise, and behavior treatment are used together. Her warm personality enables Dr. Sherard to build great friendships with her patients.

Dr. Sherard's interest in lifestyle medicine began as she worked as a volunteer at the Wildwood Lifestyle Center and Hospital located in Wildwood, Georgia, near her hometown of Chattanooga, Tennessee.

Authors' Acknowledgments

In every recipe for success, quality ingredients are necessary. One of these is creative genius. Along those lines, we are grateful to our publisher Ray Bard who accepted us as clients, and subsequently developed a love affair with The Full Plate Diet. Ray took a rather mundane topic like fiber and breathed into it freshness and vitality. He then worked tirelessly to take us far beyond what we imagined possible. We are blessed to now call him our friend. In the same category is Roy Williams—what you hold in your hands is in large part because of them.

The herbs and spices of our endeavor, what gives The Full Plate Diet flavor and substance, came from the staff of the Lifestyle Center of America. They worked daily to help us enrich this book, and our final product would not have been the same without them. LCA and their Board of Directors supported this undertaking from the beginning, and they truly are the receptacle that allowed The Full Plate Diet to be formed. We thank them deeply for the confidence and trust they have demonstrated in allowing us to be a part of this opportunity.

There are individuals who stand out for each of us. Diana wishes to thank her Mom, for raising her with a love for fiber-rich foods without realizing what a gift she bestowed. Teresa is thankful for her wonderful parents, who have been a source of continual inspiration. And Stuart has deep gratitude for Sandra, his wife and a secret ingredient in The Full Plate Diet recipe. Because of her, he was able to remain dedicated and focused. She worked behind the scenes, lending encouragement, editing skills, and priceless advice at the times they were needed the most.

Of course, we also acknowledge and give thanks to God, the creator of all health-giving, fiber-rich foods. We hope you enjoy the final product of our endeavors as much as we take pleasure in presenting it to you.

Publisher's Acknowledgments

The author team, directed by Stuart Seale, worked long and hard, making the book their number one priority. Their goal was to offer a diet that meets people where they are and guides them along a successful and rewarding path. They wanted the book to be immediately useful and reader friendly. We hope we have helped them achieve those goals. Coauthors Teresa Sherard and Diana Fleming brought unbounded enthusiasm and did tons of research, checked the grocery shelves, and made valuable contributions about the health and nutritional benefits of a high-fiber diet. Stuart, at all hours, was relentless in hammering out the concepts and details and bringing his real-world experience to bear.

Sherry Sprague brought all her managing editor skills just in time. She was traffic cop, cheerleader, and enforcer. And, she got us to the finish line on time.

Jeff Morris was an editor for the very first Bard Press book. Over the years I've come to appreciate his rare ability to retain the author's voice while editing with a sharp pencil and keen eye.

Deborah Costenbader, production editor extraordinaire, made sure details were correct and in place. Luke Torn with his eagle eye served once again as proofreader.

Gary Hespenheide, of Hespenheide Design, went beyond his usual stylish design to create a very useful and appealing book. The flexibility and patience of Gary and his team, especially Randy Miyake, allowed us to work through many variations and a demanding schedule.

Joe Pruss, our author services manager, coordinated the reader's survey, worked the booth at the big book show, and kept the operation running while I worked on the book.

Todd Sattersten contributed strategies for gaining the readers' commitment and sharing their success with others.

Montague, my son who lives in God's country, reviewed early drafts and provided valuable feedback.

Without Roy Williams there would be no book. As marketing strategist for The Lifestyle Center of America, he saw the significant weight loss of patients in the LCA intensive diabetes program. He knew LCA's mission was to reach as many people as possible—to offer them a way to change their eating lifestyle for the better. He said, "If you want to reach a large audience, take your success to the world with a diet book." CEO Sid Lloyd quickly got on board and under his able leadership gained the commitment of the LCA Board of Directors. All along the way, Chairman of the Board Dr. Franklin House gave support and encouragement that lifted our spirits and efforts. Roy stayed involved throughout, even proposing the idea for the book's title.

This is also a personal book for me. Before we signed the publishing agreement I started The Full Plate Diet. I lost 30 pounds in the first 5 months and have kept it off since. So, I know how it changes your life.

Ray Bard
Publisher

The Full Plate Diet All-Stars

Early on we sent the authors' first draft to 38 readers—a mix of ages from 15 to 85. We wanted to get their ideas about how to make The Full Plate Diet a better book. We encouraged them to be tough and talk to us straight. They did. Lots of good ideas. As we continued to develop the book, we went to them to report on our progress and to get their feedback. Many thanks to all our readers. They are indeed All-Stars.

Cameron Alexander
Linda Blackburn
Gwen Bosley
Rick Bramlett
Jason Brockwell
Amy Buckley
Dan Carnahan
Judy Carr
Ed Conway
Diana Deaton
Tamara Eaves
Tommy Emde
Amy Esqueda
Jennifer Evans
Joe Hamilton
Sue Hawkins
Kate Hendricks
Rosie Hilliard
Meg LaBorde Kuehn

Marge Lambert
Pat Miller
Hazel Nobe
Kenneth C. Nobe
Mona Ozbirn
Laura Pack
JoAnn Panke
Jerry Pruss
Kim Pruss
Peggy Pruss
Kay Roach
Cynthia Robbins
Jennie Rollins
Sara Schneider
Elmer H. Seale
Jordan Seale
Sarah Sprague
Felicia Stonedale
Ane Urquiola

Index

Photo Credits

Who We Are & Why We Care About You

The Lifestyle Center of America is a 501c3 non-profit group of people whose only mission is to improve the health and vitality of human beings around the world.

You love your life enough to be reading this book right now, so you're the person we were sent to help.

We've got all kinds of resources available to you that aren't available in bookstores. You'll find them at **www.FullPlateDiet.org**. Just look for the button marked "Resources."

Or you can call us at 877-775-2610.

Here is one of our recent publications available only from us direct—not available in retail stores.

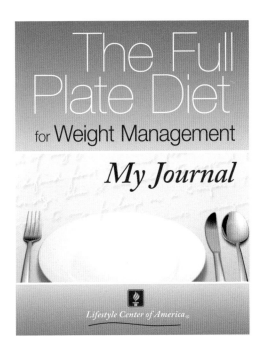

Book Order Information

To order more copies of

The Full Plate Diet
Slim Down, Look Great, Be Healthy!

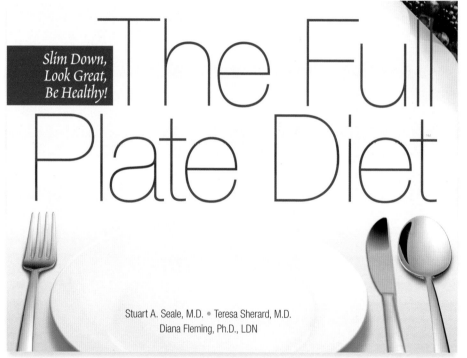

Hardcover $19.95

Visit your favorite bookstore

or

For orders of 100 or more you can also call 800-596-5480 Ext 3015

Quantity discounts available

I'm Ready!

I've read the first 3 chapters in The Full Plate Diet. I like the concept and both payoffs—losing the pounds and better natural health. I'm ready to go.

I've read and understand the 3 things I need to do in Stage One:

1. Eat more fiber foods.
2. Drink more water—at least 6 glasses a day.
3. Stop eating when I no longer feel hungry.

I'm committed to making it work for me. I see a thinner me.

_____   _____

My Name   Date

Your future is created
by what you do today,
not tomorrow.

—Robert Kiyosaki
Rich Dad, Poor Dad series

I'm Going for It!

I'm going to make some conscious changes in the way I eat that will make a big difference in how I look and feel. I'm getting slim!

The Full Plate Diet is about eating foods I like, and making sure I eat a lot more foods with fiber—fruits, vegetables, beans, and whole grains.

I'm going to eat more fiber, drink more water, and stop eating when I am not hungry.

This is a long-term, sustainable lifestyle change that will give me energy and improve my health in many ways.

Expect me to start looking slimmer soon—and know that I'll be eating more fruits, vegetables, beans, and whole grains at every opportunity.

Wish me well.

Whatever you can do or dream you can, begin it.
Boldness has genius, power, and magic in it.
Begin it now.

—Goethe

No pessimist ever discovered the secret of
the stars, or sailed to an unchartered land, or
opened a new doorway for the human spirit.

—Helen Keller

The Full Plate Diet

Shopper's Fiber Guide—Top 55 Fiber Foods

Tops Fruits

- Apples
- Bananas
- Blackberries
- Blueberries
- Guava
- Kiwis
- Mangoes
- Oranges
- Papaya
- Peaches
- Pears
- Raspberries
- Strawberries

Top Vegetables

- Avocado
- Beets
- Broccoli
- Carrots
- Corn
- Green cabbage
- Kale
- Romaine lettuce
- Spinach
- Sweet potatoes
- Tomatoes
- Zucchini

Top Beans & Peas

- Black beans
- Black-eyed peas
- Garbanzo beans
- Green beans
- Green peas
- Kidney beans
- Lentils
- Lima beans
- Navy beans
- Peas
- Pinto beans

Top Grains

- Brown rice
- Buckwheat groats
- Millet
- Oats
- Pearl barley
- Quinoa
- Rye flakes
- Wheat
- Whole-grain cornmeal
- Wild rice

Top Nuts & Seeds

- Almonds
- Brazil nuts
- Chia seeds
- Flaxseeds
- Hazelnuts (filberts)
- Peanuts
- Pecans
- Pumpkin seeds
- Sunflower seeds
- Walnuts

The Exchange

More This	**Less That***
✔ Oranges	Orange Juice
✔ Brown Rice	White Rice
✔ High-Fiber Tortillas	White Flour Tortillas
✔ Whole-Grain Bread	White Bread
✔ Almonds	Candy
✔ Apples/Bananas	Cookies
✔ Sweet Potatoes	White Potatoes
✔ Berries	Brownies
✔ Oatmeal	Eggs
✔ Fruit Smoothies	Milk Shakes
✔ Beans or Hummus Dips	Sour Cream Dip
✔ Bran Muffins	Donuts
✔ Fruit Sorbets	Ice Creams
✔ Applesauce	Pudding
✔ Beans & Salsa on Baked Potatoes	Butter & Sour Cream on Baked Potatoes

* These have little or no fiber

> The secret of getting ahead is getting started.
>
> —Mark Twain

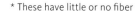

STOP

CHALLENGE

CHOOSE